FAITH BASED

FITNESS

Dr. Kenneth H. Cooper

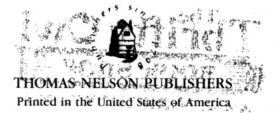

THOMAS NELSON PUBLISHERS
Printed in the United States of America

DEDICATION

To achieve harmony in my life, I have always found that I must keep God at the top, my family second, and my work third. The one person who for almost four decades has enabled me to keep my priorities right has been my beautiful wife, Millie. To recognize in some small way her wonderful, loving, and unwavering support, I dedicate this book to her.

Published in Nashville, Tennessee, by Thomas Nelson, Inc.,

Scripture quotations are from the NEW KING JAMES VERSION of the Bible. Copyright © 1979, 1980, 1982, Thomas Nelson, Inc., Publishers.

Library of Congress Cataloging-in-Publication Data

Cooper, Kenneth H.
    [It's better to believe]
    Faith based fitness : the medical program that uses spiritual
motivation to achieve maximum health and add years to your life /
Kenneth H. Cooper.
        p. cm.
    Originally published under title: It's better to believe.
    Includes bibliographical references and index.
    ISBN 0-7852-7137-6 (pbk.)
    1. Physical fitness—Religious aspects—Christianity.
2. Christian life. I. Title.
[BV4598.C66 1997]
248.4—dc21   97–19280
                                                   CIP

Printed in the United States of America

14 15 16   06 05 04

CONTENTS

ACKNOWLEDGMENTS

The preparation of a book of this magnitude requires the cooperation and support of so many people that it always frightens me to try to acknowledge them. I worry that I will leave someone out, and I know that there are many people whose names I cannot list due to space limitations. Yet despite these reservations, I must recognize those whose contributions were invaluable.

My professional literary collaborator, William Proctor, has been the key person in the organization and presentation of this book. Bill's patience was matched only by his perseverance in helping to prepare the manuscript. He has helped me in this way for the past twelve years, and so I want to say once again: another great job, Bill, and many thanks!

The person who has been central to my literary success is my friend, agent, and adviser, Herbert M. Katz. Herb started working with me in 1966 as we prepared the manuscript for the book which started it all—*Aerobics*. Since that time, he has been basically responsible for the publication of another twelve books. Although I like to think of Bill, Herb, and myself as a literary team, without Herb's wife and business partner, Nancy, nothing would be accomplished as effectively. She assures the accuracy, continuity, and readability of all my books, and her tireless efforts are most appreciated.

A relatively new member of my literary team is my editor from Thomas Nelson, Bruce Nygren. Bruce reviewed and critiqued this manuscript, as well as one of my previous books, *Antioxidant Revolution,* and he has played an important role helping to shape *Faith-Based Fitness* into its final form. Also, I wish to extend my special thanks to Thomas Nelson Vice President Kenneth Stephens for his inspiring and enthusiastic support for my work.

Keep in mind that for me, being an author is an avocation. I still practice medicine, carry a heavy patient load, and fulfill numerous other responsibilities. Organizing my patient appointments, lecture engagements, endless administrative meetings, business appointments, and book responsibilities is a very demanding, almost impossible task. There is only one person I know who can do this job and remain calm and unruffled—my secretary and administrative assistant, Harriet Guthrie. Harriet has ably and efficiently met my requirements for more than twelve years, and she is still with me! Many thanks, Harriet: You are the glue that holds my complicated life together.

Speaking of holding my life together, I must turn now to the decisive role played by my family. The fact that I have dedicated this book to my wife, Millie, speaks for itself. Yet I also want to recognize my daughter, Berkley, and son, Tyler. Not only have they tolerated the workaholic lifestyle of their father, but both have been following in his footsteps. Berkley recently completed her second marathon (and as recommended in *Antioxidant Revolution*, she is taking large doses of antioxidants daily!). Tyler, while at Baylor University, qualified and participated in the National N.C.A.A. Cross Country Championships. Thanks for the thrills, kids, and may you keep exercising and enjoy long, happy, and healthy lives.

At the Cooper Aerobics Center in Dallas, we have highly qualified specialists in a multitude of disciplines. I am constantly asking them to assist in research projects, help with patients, give lectures, and contribute to new book manuscripts. These people—who include physicians, exercise physiologists, dietitians, nutritionists, personal trainers, and administrators—have never refused to respond quickly and favorably to my requests. To list them all individually would be impossible, but let me say to the 300-plus employees who work at the Cooper Aerobics Center, a great big *thanks!*

Finally, I would be remiss if I did not thank all of those whose stories have been included in this book, including those who have allowed me to use their names. That always makes the subject matter more credible as well as more interesting. Although many of the case studies and names have been changed to protect confidentiality, the incidents described in the following pages are real events that have happened to real people—and it's quite possible that similar experiences may happen to you as well.

May all of those who have participated in this project take pride in the publication of *Faith-Based Fitness*. Without your assistance and your support, it would never been published. You are all members of my team, and I know that many readers will benefit from our efforts.

Part One

The Link between Faith and Fitness

WHY BELIEF CAN LEAD TO BETTER HEALTH AND FITNESS

You've tried and tried. But all the money you've pumped into fitness and diet books, health club memberships, cross-training shoes, and gleaming exercise equipment has gone for naught.

After countless false starts, you know better than most people that the road to the couch potato's final resting place—that easy chair in front of the TV set—is paved with good intentions. To put it bluntly, you're still overweight, soft around the middle, and likely to feel winded after running a few yards to catch a bus. Or every muscle and joint in your body seems sore and creaky the day after you play a set of tennis. Or your leg muscles start cramping after you hurry across the parking lot to avoid being late to work.

Don't feel alone. After the much-ballyhooed exercise movement peaked a few years ago—a movement, I might add, that I've been promoting with all my energy around the globe for nearly three decades—the physical condition of the average person has steadily deteriorated. According to the latest available figures from the Centers for Disease Control in Atlanta, one-third of all Americans are overweight—an increase from a fairly stable 25 percent during the period from 1960 to 1980.

Furthermore, nearly forty-eight million adults in the United States, who are otherwise healthy and able-bodied, are now officially classified as sedentary. That is, they are totally inactive. Although there are no physical or health reasons preventing them from engaging in some sort of easy-to-pursue, moderate exercise program, they somehow can't jump-start their systems to "get the juices flowing" for twenty or thirty minutes a day, three or four times a week. In short, many people can talk a good line about fitness and health, but they lack the inner drive to put their words into action.

Unfortunately, this situation is likely to become worse before it gets better. The percentage of those participating in vigorous jogging, swimming, cycling, and other endurance activities increased only from 16 percent in

1985 to 17 percent in 1991. And without adequate exercise and a reasonably healthy diet, increasing numbers of people are putting themselves at serious risk for costly medical treatments and procedures, and even possible death from cardiovascular problems, cancer, and many other diseases.

Are you in this position? You may know that on one level you really *want* to get into shape and become a vital, productive, high-energy person—one who is capable of excellence at work and of rendering maximum service to others. But you've discovered instead that you are overtired, physically soft, and disease prone.

What's the secret to bridging this gap between merely wishing you were in shape and actually getting into shape? The answer begins with belief—specifically, your deepest personal convictions about what is good and true and ultimately important about your life.

More specifically, you must take what scientists have identified as your *intrinsic* beliefs and make them an integral part of your basic approach to health and fitness.

The Scientific Side of Belief

In measuring the life-changing potential of belief, researchers have distinguished between convictions that are *extrinsic* and those that are *intrinsic.*

Extrinsic belief may include bare membership in a particular church or synagogue, the rote, mechanical recitation of a liturgy, or the intellectual affirmation of a particular set of convictions or statement of faith. The distinguishing feature of this sort of belief is that it remains in the head and never makes it to the heart. Various studies have demonstrated that these outward practices and affirmations don't have the power in themselves to improve one's spiritual status, emotional well-being, physical health—or much of anything else.

Intrinsic belief, however, is quite a different matter. It's characterized by such qualities as profound spiritual commitment, a sense of having found the ultimate meaning of life, a devotion to heartfelt prayer, and a quest for a truly transformed life. This kind of inner conviction—which may be accompanied by, but is never limited to outward, external observance—is the key to real spiritual power. Furthermore, intrinsic belief has the capacity to spark major personal enrichment in every area of life—including dramatic improvements in physical health, emotional well-being, and levels of fitness.

How Can Intrinsic Belief Benefit Your Health?

A raft of recent scientific studies has established that having deep personal convictions and values can do wonders for almost every aspect of your physical and emotional well-being. Here are some specific enhancements to health that have been linked to firm, inner commitments to moral principles, social values, God, or even oneself.

LESS DEPRESSION, SMOKING, AND ALCOHOL ABUSE

In a study of more than five hundred African-American men conducted by Wayne State University in Detroit, significant associations emerged between the participants' religious involvement and their health. The researchers identified a number of indicators of true religious commitment, including overall religiosity and church attendance. They found these were linked to various beneficial health effects, such as less depression, little or no smoking, and infrequency of alcohol consumption, according to the November 1994 issue of the *Journal of the National Medical Association.*

HEALTHIER MOTHERS AND BABIES

Maternity patients with a strong religious commitment, and their newborns, who were studied at the Department of Family Medicine, East Carolina University, had fewer medical complications than maternity patients without a religious affiliation. These results were reported in November 1994 in the *Southern Medical Journal.*

PROTECTION FROM COLON AND RECTAL CANCER

In an Australian study of patients with cancer of the colon or rectum, reported in November 1993 in the *Journal of the Royal Society of Medicine,* 715 cancer patients were compared with 727 "controls" (members of a control group) without cancer.

The researchers found that the respondents who saw themselves as most religious were less likely to have cancer than those who were not as religious. In other words, self-perceived "religiousness" was a statistically significant protective factor against the disease!

Another interesting finding in this study was that self-reported or perceived religiousness was associated with median survival times of sixty-two months. In contrast, those patients who reported themselves as "nonreligious" had a median survival time of only fifty-two months.

IMPROVED COPING WITH BREAST CANCER

A number of studies have associated a deep religious faith with an ability to cope more effectively with cancer, including breast cancer.

Researchers at the University of Texas Health Science Center at San Antonio published a study in the *Oncologocial Nurse's Forum* in September 1993 about the impact of deep faith on the condition of women with breast cancer. They found that with a group of Anglo-American patients, "intrinsic religiousness" was a strong predictor of spiritual well-being and hope—both of which are important factors for successfully coping with cancer.

A HEALTHIER EMOTIONAL BALANCE

A study at Brigham Young University in Provo, Utah, ranked participating young men and women as high, medium, or low in the quality of their personal religious commitment. Those in the *high* religious category, regardless of their religious denomination, scored highest for self-esteem, emotional maturity, and nondepression, according to the June 1993 issue of *Psychological Reports.*

REDUCED LEVELS OF STRESS

Sometimes, just believing in *yourself* can produce significant health benefits. A group of volunteer nurses working in a 2,000-bed hospital in Taiwan were under tremendous pressure on the job, and all demonstrated a lack of confidence and self-assertiveness. As part of a study that was reported in July-August 1994 in *Issues of Mental Health in Nursing,* they were divided into two groups. One group received assertiveness training (i.e., instruction in how to stand up for themselves with colleagues and superiors). The members of the other control group were put into a computer class that had no special relationship to their work problems.

The researchers found that the group that received assertiveness training—and thus learned to rely on and believe in themselves more—lowered their levels of stress significantly over a period of several weeks during which their progress was followed.

LOWER BLOOD PRESSURE AND A HEALTHIER CARDIOVASCULAR SYSTEM

A commitment to maintain significant social ties, including marriage and religious community involvements—and a willingness to act on such commitments—can have tremendous beneficial effects on health.

A study on this issue, involving more than 1,100 healthy men and women aged seventy to seventy-nine, was reported by Yale epidemiologist Lisa Berkman at a January 1995 meeting of the American Medical Association. She confirmed that strong emotional support and social ties can help lower blood pressure and enhance survival after a heart attack.

Berkman also found that significant social ties, including close friendships and family relationships, improved the levels in the brain of the chemicals norepinephrine and cortisol, which have been associated with excessive stress.

STRONGER MARRIAGE TIES

A study in the August 1993 issue of the journal *Demography* concluded that religious compatibility between spouses at the time of marriage has a large influence on marital stability. This study, which was conducted by E. L. Lehrer and C. U. Chiswick of the Economics Department of the University of Illinois at Chicago, also found that spouses of different faiths generally break up more often than those with a common faith.

A commitment to a meaningful marriage—rather than just cohabiting with a partner or remaining single—has also been linked in scientific studies to some specific health benefits. Researchers from the University of Chicago reported at conferences of the Population Association of America in April 1995 that divorced men had twice the rate of alcohol abuse as married men. Divorced women also had more problems with alcohol than their married counterparts. Other researchers at the conference said that those who live together before marriage have higher divorce rates, are more likely to be sexually disloyal, and are generally less happy than married couples.

OVERCOMING POOR FOOD HABITS—INCLUDING OVEREATING THAT LEADS TO OBESITY

The prevalence of "yo-yo" dieting—or the vicious cycle that involves losing weight and then gaining it back over and over again—is well known. Similarly, the majority of those on low-cholesterol, low-fat, or salt-restricted diets violate their regimens with alarming regularity.

A major reason for poor eating discipline is that most people have a relatively weak belief in the need for good eating—and as a result, they possess few defenses against the distractions and temptations that often get in the way of a healthy diet.

Some of the most common confessions I hear from my patients go like this:

- "I know I shouldn't be eating so much between meals, but when my stomach starts to growl, I can't help myself."
- "I know I'm eating too many saturated fats, but I often forget which foods are high in fat—and I can't carry a nutritional handbook around with me."
- "I know I should cut back on my drinking, but when I'm out with friends, well . . ."

Yet the problem most people have with sticking to a good, healthy diet goes far deeper than merely failing to abide by good intentions. The real difficulty is that they have never understood that their eating habits should reflect their deepest beliefs about life. In other words, they have failed to learn that the right kind of food can transform them into the energetic, healthy people they are meant to be. It's only with such an understanding about the connection between basic values and eating habits that a person is likely to experience lasting, beneficial dietary change.

How do you establish this all-important connection between your beliefs and your eating habits?

The first step is to gather the minimum facts you need to make an intelligent decision about smart eating. This point is reinforced by the findings of researchers in the Program in Dietetics at the University of Arkansas, as reported in the November 1994 issue of the *Journal of the Arkansas Medical Society*. They confirmed that ignorance about nutrition was directly related to poor food choices.

For example, they found that people with less than a high school education often *never* ate some of the essential items like vegetables, fruits, or milk. Also, those with less knowledge frequently chose high-fat, rather than low-fat foods. On the other hand, as the age and income level of the person increased, there was more of a tendency to pick low-fat products, as well as to consume *all* the important foods like fruits and vegetables.

The lesson is clear: First, learn all you can about the amounts and types of foods that will maximize your health and fitness. Then, recognize that adjusting your eating habits to conform with what you have learned will help you live up to your most important values and aspirations.

The Link between Faith and Fitness

Just as strong belief can produce significant benefits in other areas of health, your deepest personal convictions—including your religious faith—can become the key you've been seeking to unlock the doorway to better fitness.

I'm reminded, for instance, of one forty-three-year-old patient who went through at least four or five "false starts" in launching an exercise program. She would become very enthusiastic about fast walking, then low-impact aerobics classes, and then indoor cycling. She even went so far as to buy expensive athletic gear and equipment. But each time, after a workout or two, she gave up.

"I just can't seem to generate any enthusiasm about exercise," she said. "I'm so undisciplined."

Obviously, her problem was a lack of motivation, and so the challenge was to discover the "hot spot" in her personality that would spark a commitment that wouldn't burn out. In her case, the answer was her personal religious faith. She had been complaining of low energy levels and a feeling that she was "getting old before her time."

"I used to be able to put in several hours every weekend to help to tutor children from low-income families," she said. "But now I can hardly get out of bed on Saturday mornings."

During a relatively short discussion, she recognized that her lack of energy was directly related to her lack of exercise. She just didn't have the endurance or fitness to help the poor children who had long been her concern. Furthermore, she saw that by failing to get into shape, she was actually subverting her deepest personal values. Conversely, she realized that improving her physical condition would enable her to live more consistently within the principles of her belief system.

Now she had the key to solve her exercise problem. Whenever she was tempted not to go out for a walk or to skip an aerobics class, she always resorted to a simple routine: She would sit down for a few seconds and say a short prayer, asking for the strength to take the next step toward fulfilling her exercise commitment.

Then, she would stand up and *take* that step. Sometimes, this meant just getting into her shorts and sneakers. Sometimes, it was a matter of hopping in her car and heading for the gym. In any event, linking her beliefs to her fitness goals worked by helping her get started each day on the right path—and within a month, she was feeling more energetic and vital than she had in years.

Your beliefs are the most powerful motivational tools you have—if you can just learn how to use them. In *Faith-Based Fitness,* you'll find the proven, faith-based programs you need to achieve a healthier and more active life. Among other things, you'll learn:

- How to evaluate your personal beliefs—and ways to strengthen and use those beliefs as motivators to improve your health and fitness. A "spiritual checkup" system will be provided.
- A method to find your *Real Age*—which is determined by your actual physical condition—as opposed to your chronological age.
- How to design your own personal endurance and strength programs—and be transformed in a few months from a total couch potato into a fit, high-energy dynamo.
- Exciting ways to combine the physical and spiritual dimensions of your life, including the use of prayer and meditation in your daily workouts.
- Techniques to fine-tune your fitness efforts—so as to avoid boredom and a breakdown of discipline—by varying your activities and exercise companions.

- Ways to add many "high-velocity years" to your life, including the time you have available to devote to charitable causes and to serve others.
- The special concerns of women exercisers, who have begun to improve their energy, strength, and overall physical condition. This section will include discussions of how women can protect their knees (which are constructed differently from those of men), their backs (which are particularly vulnerable to injury), and their Achilles tendons (which may become shortened from wearing high heels).
- Practical, faith-based strategies for lowering your risk of heart disease, cancer, and a variety of other illnesses.
- A suggested philosophy of "inner food," which will give you the tools and self-confidence to select the healthiest foods at each meal and transform the way you approach what you eat.
- Practical insights from sages throughout history that suggest exciting connections between a healthy spirit and a healthy body.

By following this systematic path, you'll soon dispel any doubts you may have had about your ability to become fit. An active, energetic life will start to become a permanent reality for you. Or in the words of the prophet Isaiah: "[T]hose who wait on the LORD shall renew their strength; they shall mount up with wings like eagles, / they shall run and not be weary, / they shall walk and not faint."

I myself needed just this sort of program when I was about thirty years old. I was flabby, unfit, and well on my way to a personal medical disaster. But through a series of transforming events, I was able to develop from a classic overweight, out-of-shape blob into my current identity—the Father of Aerobics, as I have been called by the popular press.

2

A PERSONAL ADVENTURE WITH THE POWER OF BELIEF

When I was a schoolboy in the community of Putnam City, Oklahoma, a suburb of Oklahoma City, I didn't always make a conscious connection between my faith and my commitment to athletics. But these two threads in my personality intertwined rather naturally as I studied and admired the lives of vigorous, energetic Old and New Testament figures in our local Baptist church—and at the same time increased my *own* vigor and energy by participating to the hilt in organized sports.

My faith began to grow after I was baptized at the age of nine. For as long as I can remember, I attended Sunday school classes and our church's morning and evening worship services. Biblical principles and illustrations became as much a part of my life as breathing.

I can still remember offering short prayers every so often as I ran the mile and a half to school every morning—roadwork that was part of my training for track and cross country. In the afternoon, I participated in basketball or football practice with my high school teams. Then I'd jog the mile and a half home again. This rigorous exercise routine seemed an essential part of what God wanted me to do with my life at that point. I never questioned the importance of my athletic activities, any more than I questioned my academic demands or the need to attend church.

My father, who was a prominent dentist in our city, did raise some strong objections to my heavy sports involvement. His main concern was that he thought I would develop an "athletic heart" from such a vigorous regimen. This was a commonly held myth subscribed to by many people in those days, even medical professionals. He argued that if I continued to work out so much, my heart would first become unnaturally large, then turn to fat, and finally become vulnerable to a fatal heart attack.

Now, of course, we know such fears are groundless, but I had to listen to his worries regularly when I was at home. Dad felt so strongly about the issue that, even though he didn't forbid me to participate in sports, he never attended any of my games or track meets. He even tried his best to get me to cut back on the level of my activities.

Finally, I did drop football, perhaps in part because of my father's fears. But the main thing that bothered me was the possibility of serious, permanent injury to my bones or joints.

Outside events forced me into a decision. I was playing wide receiver at the time, and after suffering a series of hard hits to my knees during my junior year, I made an appointment with the coach. I told him I thought I should quit because of the possibility of a debilitating injury that could end my basketball and track careers. He wasn't happy about the idea, but he understood. So I abandoned football to concentrate on my other sports.

The decision turned out to be just the right thing for me. I was selected for the All-State Oklahoma basketball team, I won the state championship in the mile run—and athletic scholarship offers began to pour in. One recruiter even tried to bribe me by attempting to stick a $20 bill in my running shoes. I was so naive that I didn't have any idea what was going on. Fortunately, I didn't have to get into a discussion with the man: When I saw him poking around my shoe, I asked rather loudly, "What are you doing?" and he beat a hasty retreat with his money.

Before the end of my senior year, I settled on a track scholarship to the University of Oklahoma. My goal in those days was to run the mile in the Olympics—a dream I never realized because I failed to lower my time below 4:18 in college. Still, even as I prepared to enter medical school following my college graduation, it seemed that vigorous exercise would always be a part of my life. I couldn't imagine otherwise.

But after I embarked on my medical studies at the University of Oklahoma, everything changed. My physical condition began to go downhill because, like many other former high school and college athletes, I no longer had access to the supportive, motivating environment of a team. There was no coach to tell me when to show up for practice or how many miles to run. There were no teammates to provide camaraderie and spur me on with friendly competition. In short, I had lost all my outside reinforcement to keep exercising—and I saw no real reason to pursue an independent fitness program on my own. I completely lacked any inner motivation.

Even my religious faith, which had fit so naturally into my athletic activities in school, somehow didn't seem relevant to my current physical condition. I didn't even think it was important enough to pray about the matter. Instead, I pushed sports and exercise out of my mind entirely and concentrated primarily on doing well in medical school. It didn't dawn on me that maybe my faith *demanded* that I do my best to keep my body in good shape.

I paid dearly for this oversight. By the time I had finished medical school, completed my internship, and spent a few years as a doctor in the U.S. Army, my weight had ballooned up from my ideal athletic level of 165 pounds to an all-time high of 204 in my late twenties—forty pounds of excess baggage to carry around! Also, as a result of the inactivity and extra weight, my blood pressure had crept up so that I had actually become a borderline hypertensive.

The abuse of my body didn't end here. To meet the demands of medical school and my early medical practice, I had fallen into the habit of limiting myself to three or four hours of sleep a night—a practice that kept my stress levels sky-high and undercut my efficiency and the clarity of my thinking. My technique for staying awake was to eat, and that meant downing any kind of junk food I could put my hands on. In effect, I was mainlining artery-clogging fats into my blood vessels.

As a consequence of this neglect, a major health crisis started brewing in my life. In 1960, when I was just going on thirty, I transferred from the Army to the Air Force. I had just married my wife, Millie, and I can still remember a conversation we had as I stretched out in exhaustion on our sofa at a Texas Air Force base where we were stationed. Hardly able to move after a relatively moderate day of work, I told her, "I'm getting fatter every minute, and I'm dying of mental stagnation."

Millie was nice enough not to agree with my self-evaluation—but she didn't disagree either. I'm sure she wondered what kind of a dull, lethargic character she had chosen for a husband. While we were engaged, I had regaled her with stories of my past athletic exploits and future career aspirations, including my desire to qualify in a medical specialty and maybe even become a physician-astronaut. As she saw me lying inert on that couch, I suspect she was puzzled about what exactly had happened to the ambitious guy who had courted her. I know *I* was wondering what had gone wrong. I realized I needed to change my life, but somehow I lacked the inner drive to take even the first necessary steps toward personal transformation.

Then, something happened to get my attention. I was invited to go waterskiing with some friends and was told that there would be an opportunity to do some slaloming. I hadn't been on water skis in about eight years, but when I was younger, I had been pretty good at the sport—and had successfully negotiated a number of demanding slalom courses. So I figured this might be just the opportunity I needed to embark on a more active way of life and lose some of the rolls of fat that had accumulated around my middle.

When we arrived at the lake, I was the first at the dock, and I could hardly wait for the speedboat to get warmed up. "I'll try the slalom course first thing," I told the boat operator.

"Wouldn't you like to try one short practice swing around the lake, just to get used to the skis again?" the operator asked.

"No, I'm ready for the slalom."

I was still feeling supremely confident when the boat lunged forward and I felt the familiar tug of the line, which pulled me to an upright position on my skis. But a few minutes later, I knew I was heading for trouble. Waterskiing isn't an aerobic or endurance activity in the same way that jogging, swimming, and cycling are. But the sport does require plenty of muscle stamina and strength, especially in the thighs, stomach, shoulders, and arms—and these were physical qualities that I sorely lacked.

The extra forty pounds I was carrying, plus my greatly diminished muscle tone and endurance, were a formula for disaster. As I struggled at high speed around the slalom buoys, I thought I might collapse any moment. My legs, shoulders, and arms grew tired and then *dead* tired. Next, the pain set in. More parts of my body than I could count felt as though they were coming unglued. Before long, everything started to go numb—and my breath came in short, agonizing gasps.

Somehow I made it back to the beach without falling off the skis, but then I stumbled out of the water onto the bank and tumbled to the ground in a heap. Nausea swept over me. My heart rate soared so high that I knew it was hammering away at close to 250 beats per minute—when the maximum rate should have been 190 to 200.

Though I wasn't entirely lucid, my medical training kicked in automatically: I was able to diagnose myself as suffering from supraventricular tachycardia, an exceptionally high heart beat that *must* be reduced rather quickly if serious consequences are to be averted. I'm not ashamed to say I was *scared*—really terrified. I wasn't ready to die.

Fortunately, after I had rested quietly on that lake bank for several minutes, my heart rate decreased. After five or six minutes, it was down to about 120 beats per minute. Thirty minutes later, the rate was down to my normal resting rate of 60 to 70 beats per minute. But even though the crisis had passed, I had heard the wake-up call.

"What have I done to myself?" I asked over and over, as I watched the other skiers going through their paces. "I've really gone to pot—and I've got to do something about it!"

I realized that I had no one to blame but myself for my close brush with medical emergency. I also started to understand, perhaps for the first time, that my body was truly a "temple of God," but a temple I had allowed to fall into sad disrepair. It was clearly up to *me* to keep that temple in shape if I hoped to live a complete life and fulfill the plans God had for my life.

This "fitness conversion" was all I needed to get on the right track. I immediately resolved to start exercising several times a week, and because running was the sport I knew best, I focused on that. At first, I could only run for a few hundred yards before I had to stop and walk to catch my breath.

It was slow, hard work, especially for the first two to three weeks. But I kept at it, and the commitment paid off. At the end of six months, I was running two to three miles at a stretch, five or six days a week. This exercise, plus eating a more moderate diet, enabled me to lose more than thirty of the extra pounds I had put on. Also, my blood pressure readings declined to the normal range.

At the same time—and I don't believe this was any coincidence—some other loose ends in my life began to fall into place. I became more sensitive to God's presence in my life and to the control he was exercising over my destiny and career, including my acceptance as a graduate student at the Harvard School of Public Health. While in Boston, I became intrigued by the possibility of using preventive medicine techniques, such as exercise, to improve the health of others and reduce their risk for various diseases. In particular, I began investigating the use of stress testing to check a person's capacity to consume oxygen during vigorous exercise. This research was one of my first steps toward establishing standards for individual fitness levels and developing systematic conditioning programs, such as what later developed into my internationally recognized aerobics points system.

My career as a preventive medicine specialist really began at this point. And my personal interest in fitness intensified as I accepted a challenge by a colleague to train for the Boston Marathon.

An Ultimate Test for a New Fitness Believer

"You want to explore the benefits of endurance exercise?" one of my Harvard colleagues asked. "A marathon is the *ultimate* endurance experience."

In those relatively early days of distance running, a marathon was an exotic event—a race covering slightly more than twenty-six miles was considered by many to be at best eccentric, and maybe even slightly insane. A year earlier, when I had been bemoaning my sad physical condition, my lack of drive in my career, and my general malaise about life, I couldn't have imagined in my wildest fantasies that I would ever even *see* a marathon, much less participate in one.

But I had come a long way since that waterskiing fiasco. Now, I wanted to see just how much progress I had made, and the marathon was a worthy test. So for several months, I ran mile after mile during the free time I had available—and I must admit, there wasn't too much. I was simultaneously studying for German and Russian qualifying exams, pursuing my exercise research, and taking an extra load of courses because I thought I might want to go on and get a second doctorate in exercise physiology. Millie learned what it was like to become a runner's widow during that phase of our marriage.

Finally, the big day arrived in the spring of 1962. Crowded up close to about 150 other participants, I found myself waiting tensely for the crack of the gun at the starting line. Though a far cry from today's Boston Marathon, with its thousands of participants, the classic race was still an awe-inspiring event, with world-class distance runners rubbing shoulders with novices like me.

The first five or six miles weren't so bad, but then things began to get rough. I developed some serious blisters about seven miles into the race, but I kept on going. For me, the Boston competition was an important test. I had been working out intensively—sometimes running as far as twenty straight miles in one session—and I knew I had made tremendous progress in improving my physical condition. Now, I wanted to see just how far I had come, and I wasn't about to let some annoying little blisters stop me.

The miles rolled on slowly under my feet—ten, fifteen, eighteen. Then, at about the twenty-mile mark, I hit the proverbial "wall," the physiologic obstacle that distance runners dread. The glycogen, or sugar, stores in my muscles had become totally depleted, and I started to burn fat to provide the energy required to keep on going. When the body's metabolism shifts to using fat, the muscles start to hurt—*bad*. My legs felt like lead, as the calves, knees, and thighs literally filled with pain. My feet were in such agony from the burst blisters that they began to throb and then go numb, to the point that I almost couldn't feel them at all.

Finally, half walking and half stumbling, I crossed the finish line in 101st place, three hours and fifty-four minutes after I had started the race. Although Millie was waiting there for me, most of the other spectators had left. The judges were still recording times—but only because of Millie's cajoling and pleading. They had been ready to pack up and leave at three-and-a-half hours, but Millie had said, "You can't quit! I don't want Ken to arrive and find no one here!"

The judges tried arguing with her, but you don't argue with Millie when she sets her mind on something. They finally gave up and resigned themselves to waiting for me to show up. As a result, I was listed as the last official finisher in the 1962 event.

Although it was considered a great honor in those days just to finish a marathon, any accolades or glory escaped me at the time. I was so exhausted I could barely drag myself over to the makeshift runners' medical post at the old Lenox Hotel, where I had to wait in line to see one of the foot doctors who were treating those with injuries. I could hardly stand on my feet, which had turned into a bloody mess.

When I finally got to see a podiatrist, he took one look at my feet and said, "Son, when did you get those blisters?"

"I had those seven miles into the race," I said.

"Son," he replied, "you don't need a foot doctor. You need a head doctor."

For the next day or so, as I tried to hobble about on my hurting feet, I wondered whether he might be right. Maybe I had been overdoing this fitness business. Then the pain subsided, and the magnitude of my personal achievement hit me. In a little over a year I had gone from being the consummate couch potato to passing an ultimate fitness test—completing a marathon. The next year, I entered the race again and registered another personal milestone by breaking the three-and-a-half-hour mark. I placed ninety-eighth overall—and this time my wife didn't have to talk the judges into waiting around so that I could become an official finisher.

What message might my experience have for you? Just this: If I could make this kind of progress, given my poor "before" condition, then you can as well. It doesn't matter how young or old you are. The secret to success is to find some powerful motivation to get you started and keep you going. Somehow, you have to become convinced that achieving good health and fitness is essential to transform you into the kind of person you're meant to be. In short, you have to understand what it really means to believe that your body, like your mind and spirit, has a divinely ordained destiny—a purpose that *must* be fulfilled if you are to develop into a complete human being.

What Exactly Do I Mean by "Believe"?

Let me begin these reflections on the meaning of belief with a word of caution: When I talk about the kind of belief that can revolutionize your health, I'm *not* referring to some sort of financial substitute for true religious faith. Rather, the belief required for a "fitness conversion" involves a conviction about your body and health that should be an outgrowth of your basic spiritual worldview. Any focus on physical conditioning must always be kept subordinate to the more comprehensive, eternal beliefs of the spirit. Or as it says in the Bible, "Bodily exercise profits a little, but godliness is profitable for all things" (1 Tim. 4:8).

Those who allow their fitness programs to become all-consuming will soon find that other essential values, such as maintaining strong personal and family relationships, begin to crumble. For example, there was the marathon enthusiast who left his wife and small children alone most eve-

---

A Journey from the Outside to the Inside

In her *Gift from the Sea*, Anne Morrow Lindbergh, in contemplating a seashell, discovers a profound connection between the inner and outer life:

> *Simplification of outward life is not enough. It is merely the outside. But I am starting with the outside. I am looking at the outside of a shell, the outside of my life—the shell. The complete answer is not to be found on the outside, in an outward mode of living. This is only a technique, a road to grace. The final answer, I know, is always inside. But the outside can give a clue, can help one to find the inside answer.*
>
> —from Anne Morrow Lindbergh, *Gift from the Sea*
> (New York: Random House/Vintage Books, 1978), p. 35.

Lessons from Anne Morrow Lindbergh:

- The physical dimension of our lives, which is always a primary focus during exercise, should never become an end in itself. Rather, our bodies should open the door to deeper, more profound inner experiences.
- Listen to your body, which can give you clues or insights relating to what is happening in your inner nature.

---

nings as he trained for two to three hours after work. His marriage ended after he had completed his third year of intensive distance racing. Just as tragically, his children hardly knew him. They were almost always in bed by the time he arrived home after a workout.

Similarly, there was the "tennis nut," who played at his club several evenings a week. Somehow this marriage managed to survive—but only because his wife laid down an ultimatum: "Either you cut your tennis back to one evening a week, or you accept the consequences." He didn't ask what those consequences might be. But he took the warning seriously and shifted his playing to the mornings before work and to weekend hours that wouldn't interfere with family time.

So you should first understand that good health and fitness are only a *part* of life, not the be-all and end-all of your existence. If you believe otherwise, you're heading for trouble, if not tragedy.

At the same time, I don't want to downplay in any way the significance of improving your physical condition. The weight of the scientific evidence and most clinical findings, including my own experiences with my patients, show clearly that better health and fitness are essential to a full and effective life. Unless disease or disability dictates otherwise, your body *must* work properly if you hope to enjoy the energy you need to handle life's mental and spiritual challenges.

But to get started and then keep on going require more than mere intellectual assent or lip service. You have to move beyond just saying, "Hey, getting in shape sounds like a really good idea!" Or, "You've convinced me, Ken—maybe I'll try that some day." Or, "When my schedule opens up, I'll definitely consider starting some sort of program, but I really don't have time to include regular exercise in my life right now."

Your schedule will never magically "open up" unless you understand that your basic faith *demands* that you take good care of your body. And that means making a firm commitment that will get you off your backside and launch you on a life-changing program—such as the one I'm suggesting in *Faith-Based Fitness*. Specifically, there are two stages or steps that lead to the kind of belief that has transformed my physical condition and the condition of thousands of other sedentary people I've worked with over the years.

STAGE #1: A LIFE-CHANGING BELIEF BEGINS WITH AN INITIAL LEAP OF FAITH

Somehow, you have to decide the time has arrived for you to take a plunge into unknown waters. You must be willing to gamble a little time and effort to see if there just may indeed be some significant benefits that accompany a more active life.

You don't need a comprehensive fitness plan at this point, and you certainly shouldn't expect to have all the answers. You just need to be willing to step out and trust the many responsible people who are assuring you that caring for your body will make you a more effective, happier, and healthier person.

Plenty of preventive medicine and fitness professionals, including myself, will tell you that getting in shape will give you more energy, better health, and greater protection against various diseases. It's incontrovertible from research we've done at the Cooper Institute for Aerobics Research, as well as at other research centers, that becoming even *moderately* fit will dramatically reduce your risk of getting cancer, heart disease, and a host of other dangerous diseases. Spiritual seers have also added their strong endorsement to the importance of caring for your body. No less an authority than the apostle Paul has said, "Do you not know that your body is the temple of the Holy Spirit . . . ? For you were bought at a price; therefore glorify God in your body. . . ."

But most likely, despite the assurances of such an array of experts, you will still harbor some serious doubts about whether an exercise and diet program is really worth the effort. Yet that's what faith is all about. Despite your fears, your intellectual reservations, and perhaps a touch of complacency, a bold leap into the unknown can allow you to test the waters to see if *maybe* the promises you've heard are indeed true.

Don't wait for a health crisis to strike, as I did. You may not be so lucky. Make your initial move *now*—and prepare to watch your own fitness adventure unfold.

**STAGE #2: BELIEF IN YOUR BODY'S POWER GROWS
GRADUALLY THROUGH PERSONAL DISCIPLINE**

Spiritual giants don't reach their full stature overnight. Similarly, as far as your physical progress is concerned, you can't hop from being totally sedentary one day to being a marathoner the next. If you try, you'll fail. Instead, after you take that first leap of faith, it's necessary to embark on a disciplined program, which can gradually and safely turn your new, untested beliefs into a long-term reality.

Clearly, belief in the sense I'm describing it doesn't involve just *saying* you believe in the potential benefits of fitness. It requires *doing* something about it—throwing your whole self into a fitness regimen, a program like the one I'm proposing in *Faith-Based Fitness*.

When I started my own physical comeback at age thirty, I really didn't quite know what I was doing or where I would eventually end up. Without any tested program to follow, I just began by a combination of walking and jogging for relatively short distances. As my muscles toned up and my endurance increased, I stayed out for somewhat longer outings. Finally, I began to run for the entire workout, first for twenty minutes, then thirty, then forty.

Remember, it required six months for me to lose my excess weight, lower my blood pressure, and get back into fairly decent condition. Then it took *another* six months before I was ready to start training for the marathon. Today, more than thirty years later, I've logged nearly 27,000 miles of jogging, and countless additional miles of fast walking, cycling, and other demanding endurance activities such as snow skiing and mountain climbing. This ongoing, active lifestyle has only been possible because my early, rudimentary beliefs in the importance of exercise deepened with experience into absolute certainty. Actually, after only a month or two of regular endurance activity, I couldn't imagine returning to my sedentary way of life. And now, decades later, I still can't imagine it.

I've designed the programs in this book so that you can tap the power of your own beliefs to reap the full benefits of exercise—not for just a week, or a month, or a year, but for a lifetime. In many ways, your physical conditioning program should parallel your personal spiritual journey. So now, let's consider in more detail why it's truly better for you to believe—and how you can strengthen and use your beliefs to maximize your energy levels, stave off illness, and live as long as God has designed you to live.

3

IT'S TIME FOR A
SPIRITUAL CHECKUP

I've always been a strong advocate of the need for regular *physical* check-ups by your doctor—and the same is true of your *spiritual* health. There's no such thing as benign neglect of the soul. Frequent examination and nurturing of the inner life are absolutely essential. Otherwise, the growth and deepening of your personal belief system will cease. And when your basic beliefs begin to deteriorate, the spark that keeps you motivated to exercise may also be extinguished.

That's what almost happened to me in 1974, a few years after my first book, *Aerobics,* became an international bestseller. I had begun to be in great demand as a speaker and advocate of the fitness movement, and I was also inundated with new patients who were interested in pursuing a program of preventive medicine. Before the onset of these overwhelming demands on my time, I had succeeded fairly well in keeping my priorities in order: God first, family second, work third, and physical fitness fourth. Although my Christian beliefs helped me approach my life in this way, I now found things were becoming topsy-turvy and generally unbalanced. Work had crept up to the top of the list, my family was at the bottom, my spiritual life had almost completely dried up—and my emotional condition and physical health were not in the best shape.

I had stopped praying regularly, reading the Bible, or even thinking much about God. It wasn't that I was having any particular doubts about his existence. I just didn't seem to have time to nurture my inner life, and simultaneously I was also finding it harder to schedule a good workout.

Although I was still trying to maintain a regular exercise routine, the workouts, when I could fit them in, seemed to leave me exhausted or unsatisfied. In the past, a good run, scheduled consistently late every afternoon, would energize me and enable me to keep going at high velocity well into the evening. But now my exercise sessions had become more sporadic. Also, my energies were sapped by many worries, including countless decisions about how to allocate my time among speaking, writing, seeing patients, and serving as administrator of the fledgling Aerobics Center and Cooper Clinic in Dallas.

Then, I got a spiritual wake-up call from Cliff Barrows, the songleader and master of ceremonies for the evangelistic crusades of Billy Graham. He asked me to speak on the platform at Graham's next big meeting, which was scheduled for Rio de Janeiro in October of 1974.

"We want you to speak at the meeting," Barrows said, referring to a talk that would include a description of my own spiritual journey and the way my faith interacted with my work in fitness and preventive medicine.

"I'll have to think about it," I told him, but I proceeded to put any thought about Billy Graham or my spiritual life completely out of my mind.

Then, about six weeks before the crusade, Cliff called again. "I'm sending you a ticket to Rio," he said.

That made me angry because I thought he was applying too much pressure. "I can't go—there is no way I can go to Rio," I said, and hung up the phone.

Although I was counseling a patient at the time, I completely forgot about him as disturbing emotions welled up: first anger, then anxiety, then fear. It never crossed my mind to pray about what I should do. Instead, I sank deeper and deeper into spiritual and emotional turmoil. There was renewed despair about my father, who had just died. Also, I worried about an encephalitis epidemic that I knew had just hit Brazil—and I wondered if my refusal to speak at the Graham rally had anything to do with being afraid that I might get the disease or even die if I went down there.

Perspiration poured down my face—evidence of the battle that was going on inside. It was a classic anxiety attack. I must have seemed to be on the verge of some sort of personal health crisis because my patient asked, "Are you all right, Dr. Cooper?"

That brought me back to reality, and I quickly assured him I was all right, even though I wasn't. I managed to get through administering my patient's exam and then shut the door and told my assistant to hold any further patients or calls for a few minutes. I knew I was in the middle of some sort of major turning point, and I was convinced that if I didn't resolve it fairly quickly, I could be heading for big trouble.

In some ways, I felt almost as though I had gone from heaven to hell during the past few years. My dreams of helping countless people through aerobic fitness programs were being realized, and my career as a leader in preventive medicine was well under way. But in the midst of this success, something had been lost. God was no longer a part of my life. I knew enough about myself to understand that the dislocation I was feeling deep inside was a sign that all was not well on the spiritual front. Once again, God was trying to get my attention.

Then a kind of mental picture flashed before me, a scene of what I could expect if I continued on my present course: I was living a life apart from God, and I even sensed I might be on the verge of some sort of catastrophe involving my children, or my wife, or my marriage, or my own health. A preoccupation with death—and serious questions about how well I had prepared myself for it—gripped me. Yet there was a way out. I didn't have to continue on my present self-centered path. Instead, I could choose to reorder my priorities and begin to honor God again.

I didn't understand everything that was happening to me, but I did know that the right thing was to reverse my decision on the Billy Graham meeting. So I picked up the phone and called Cliff Barrows.

"Something just happened to me," I told him. "I don't know exactly what it all means, but I'll be there."

When I put the phone down, my feelings of despondency and confusion were replaced by a calm certainty, a "peace that passes understanding." I knew from past experience that when I was in tune with God, there was a contentment that couldn't be explained in human terms. That's what I felt at that moment.

In the October rally in Rio, I spoke to an estimated 240,000 people about the relationship between spiritual and physical fitness. Relying on my own journey of faith—which I freely admitted had been characterized by a number of ups and downs—I told the crowd that I had recently become more convinced than ever that each of us is designed to be a flesh-and-blood temple of God. Our charge on this earth is to serve Christ and our fellow man, to exercise our gifts and talents to the maximum—and to care for all the assets God has given us, including our bodies. Solid spiritual convictions, I emphasized, will lead naturally to invigorating and enjoyable physical activities and improved conditioning.

Even before I made this trip with Billy Graham, I was known in Brazil as a kind of fitness guru. Many Brazilians had already studied and applied my aerobics programs, and they even called their fitness runs "doing a Cooper." But few of them knew of my religious beliefs or my personal history of exploring the connections between spirituality and fitness.

But even though the actual trip to Rio and the chance to share my faith on the platform with Dr. Graham were exhilarating, the really significant spiritual breakthrough for me was my decision to go in the first place. In fact, I now regard this choice as the single most important event in my adult life. I don't believe I could have gone on to write my other books, build the Cooper Institute for Aerobics Research into an international center for the scientific study of fitness, or achieve anything else without the transformation that occurred in me after I elected to follow God on this occasion.

I was certainly angry at Cliff Barrows when he called the second time to prod me into giving the talk. But I'll also always be grateful that he had the courage and patience to overlook my bad mood and resistance and keep the opportunity open. In retrospect, I can see that my big mistake was that I failed to give myself a periodic spiritual checkup. I was growing weaker and weaker in my beliefs, to the point that I was in danger of making some big mistakes, including a neglect of spiritual matters, my family, and my health. I've since learned that you don't have to wait for some emergency to get your inner being in order. All it takes is periodically posing a few key questions to yourself and then answering them honestly.

Here's a distillation of some of the most important questions that have helped me keep a close watch on my own spiritual status—and at the same time assess my ability to use my beliefs to reinforce my personal fitness program. Try asking them of yourself, and see if you feel more motivated to improve your conditioning and your health. Suggestions for scoring your answers to these questions are included at the end of the checkup.

The Spiritual Checkup

QUESTION #1: DO I BELIEVE MY BODY IS GOOD AND WORTHY OF BEING TREATED AS A CREATION OF GOD?

The first step in linking your beliefs to a fitness program is to recognize the Judeo-Christian assumption about the basic goodness of the physical world. It all begins in the book of Genesis, which makes this statement just after the creation had been finished: "Then God saw everything that He had made, and indeed it was very good." The same view is echoed by Paul in his first letter to Timothy: "For every creature of God is good. . . ."

Yet I've encountered many Christians and Jews in my medical practice who ignore these biblical injunctions. Some actually believe their bodies are completely *bad*. They may hear from their ministers or rabbis that certain sexual practices, moral habits, or other harmful activities are wrong. But then they carry these valid teachings one step too far and mistakenly conclude that *all* functions and features of the body are basically negative.

Others are more subtle in their rejection of their bodies. They believe, quite rightly, that the spiritual dimensions of their lives are of supreme importance. But then they proceed to the assumption that their physical beings are unimportant and may be neglected with impunity. They fail to understand that their spiritual lives—including the values and relationships they hold so dear—are closely connected with the condition of their bodies. If the body begins to break down, the person may lack the endurance and

---

Socrates on Exercise

The wandering Greek philosopher Socrates, who taught Plato and other great thinkers in the late fifth century B.C., was physically powerful and robust. He served tough stints as a foot soldier in the Athenian infantry and spent much of his later life walking around Greek towns and countryside, as he advocated his philosophical positions. According to Plato, he typically wore only one single, simple garment regardless of the season, and usually went barefoot, even in the dead of winter.

Socrates believed in the importance of striking a balance between training the body and the mind, as this interchange between him and a student, Glaucon, shows:

Socrates: *Have you noticed how a lifelong devotion to physical exercise, to the exclusion of anything else, produces a certain type of mind? Just as a neglect of it produces another type? One type tends to be tough and uncivilized, the other soft and over-sensitive, and . . .*

Glaucon: *Yes, I have noticed that excessive emphasis on athletics produces a pretty uncivilized type, while a purely literary and academic training leaves a man with less backbone than is decent.*

Socrates: *It is the energy and initiative in their nature that may make them uncivilized. If you treat it properly it should make them brave, but if you overstrain it, it turns them tough and uncouth, as you would expect.*

Glaucon: *I agree.*

Socrates: *The philosophic temperament, on the other hand, is gentle; too much relaxation may produce an excessive softness, but if it is treated properly the result should be civilized and humane.*

—trans. by H. D. P. Lee from Plato, The Republic
(Baltimore: Penguin Books, 1955, 1961), p. 153.

Lessons from Socrates:

- Focusing on your body to the exclusion of your spirit will make you something less than human.
- Focusing on your mind to the exclusion of your body will hamper your overall endurance and strength.
- Always strive to balance physical, mental, and spiritual exercise.

---

energy required to serve others, stay in a good mood, or even spend extended periods in prayer.

Barbara, a thirty-five-year-old legal secretary, had become seriously obese—nearly fifty pounds above her ideal weight. Her body fat registered 35 percent, well above the 21 percent it should have been. Also, she was almost completely sedentary, and blood tests revealed that she was showing signs of early diabetes.

The greatest satisfaction Barbara got out of life was to work several nights a week and several hours on weekends with a volunteer group from her church that counseled poor people about jobs and low-cost housing opportunities. But Barbara admitted that, because of her packed daily schedule, she mostly grabbed hamburgers, french fries, milk shakes, and other junk food for her evening meal. Also, she felt she had no time to engage in any sort of exercise—other than walking from her car to her law office or the counseling center. With her exclusive focus on the good she wanted to accomplish in the world, she had become blinded to the physical support systems she needed to enable her to carry out her chosen tasks effectively.

"In the last few months, I've found that I'm always feeling tired," Barbara said. "I can't concentrate well at work or in my conversations with the people I'm counseling. It's gotten so bad I often fall asleep when I'm trying to pray."

Because of her firm Christian convictions, it was easy to show Barbara that God was really concerned about her health and physical vigor. She had never before considered that perhaps her lack of energy might be linked to her poor physical condition, but now she understood clearly that there was indeed a connection. Barbara immediately resolved to take the necessary steps to improve her fitness and her health—and to enhance her efficiency at work, her spiritual life, and her ability to serve others. After learning more about what exercise and a better diet could do for her, she knew that God wanted her to walk for twenty minutes four times a week, and also that there were certain high-fat foods and desserts that he wanted her to avoid.

It's relatively easy to forget or ignore a fitness program if you assume you're trying to maintain discipline all by yourself. But if you believe, as Barbara did, that God is always available to guide and care for you, it's much harder to push your program out of your mind. Every time she deviated from her new convictions about the importance of exercise and food, she sensed she was stepping outside of God's plan for her life—and usually she returned to her regimen.

Within six months—about the length of time it took me to get back into shape myself—Barbara had dropped most of her extra weight and was down to 25 percent body fat; her blood tests were normal; and she had plenty of energy to pursue all her interests. Like many of my other patients, she had learned through experience that it really is better to believe that your body is worthy of care and attention.

QUESTION #2: DO I BELIEVE I HAVE A PERSONAL RESPONSIBILITY TO HELP *PREVENT* THE ONSET OF DISEASE?

In 1993, when he was fifty-nine years old, Kirk Fordice, the first Republican governor of Mississippi in 118 years, came to me for a physical exam. As part of his checkup, he was given a PSA blood test, which is designed to indicate the presence of prostate cancer. His result was an extremely high 15. (A normal reading should have been about 4 or lower.)

"This is cancer unless somehow we can prove the test is wrong," I said.

Fordice was deeply concerned, and initially he preferred that news about the disease be kept confidential. Of course, we honored his request. He went through a series of additional tests, including biopsies, and the diagnosis of prostate cancer was confirmed. Surgery was scheduled, but before the operation was performed, Governor Fordice called Senator Robert Dole for counsel. Dole said, "If you tell your constituency that you have cancer, lives may be saved," because others might be encouraged to have prostate exams.

So Fordice did go public before surgery. He recommended on television that every man in the state of Mississippi over the age of fifty should have a urological exam, including the PSA blood test. The response was immediately and overwhelmingly positive. Hundreds called in to say they were scheduling physical exams, and many malignancies were detected.

As for Fordice, his operation revealed that the cancer had been caught before it had spread beyond the prostate, and it took him only a few weeks to recover from the procedure. When he returned to his office, there was more good news. Several letters that were waiting for him carried the same message: The writers said that the governor's decision to go public with his cancer had probably saved their lives.

Clearly, Governor Kirk Fordice's belief in the possibility of prevention had two important effects:

- His commitment to a regular physical exam had enabled me to order the test that detected his prostate cancer—and probably saved his life.
- His courage in promoting prevention among his constituents resulted in the saving of countless other lives.

If you believe that you have the power to take steps to prevent disease in your own life—and believe me, you *do* have this power—you're well on your way to forming the inner commitment that is required to achieve better health, improved fitness, and a longer life.

QUESTION #3: DO I BELIEVE I POSSESS A NATURAL INNER POWER TO PROMOTE THE HEALING OF DISEASE?

Our minds have been endowed with an incredible capacity to affect the functioning and overall health of our bodies. When stresses overwhelm us, our emotions and bodies begin to break down; but when we develop effective strategies to handle stress, our capacity to maintain our health increases dramatically.

It's long been known that unresolved inner turmoil will lead to serious emotional problems, such as deep anxiety and depression, as well as to various physical illnesses. Yet when those inner problems are resolved, health returns to the rest of the system.

Take King David, who wrote nearly three thousand years ago in Psalm 32:3–4 that "my bones grew old / through my groaning all the day long. / For day and night Your hand was heavy upon me; / my vitality was turned into the drought of summer." Yet David said that he eliminated his inner turmoil by confessing certain sins that were weighing him down. As a result, he received God's forgiveness, his health returned, and he went on to experience great joy.

In our own day, a number of researchers have established that keeping the mind calm and balanced by relying on a firm personal belief system will have a healthful effect on the body. Dr. Herbert Benson, a professor at the Harvard Medical School, has identified what he calls the "Faith Factor" in physical and emotional healing. In his *Beyond the Relaxation Response,* he defines this Faith Factor as a means of natural healing that is made possible by the interaction of two forces: 1) a strong personal belief system that accepts the importance of caring for the body, and 2) the practice of prayer and meditation as part of those beliefs.

More specifically, Benson has found that those patients who have firm religious or philosophical convictions, and who practice regularly the disciplines of meditative prayer, tend to have the most success in healing certain health conditions. These include reducing high blood pressure, relieving headaches and backaches, and overcoming mental depression and other health problems.

It's long been known that relaxation techniques—such as prayer or meditation accompanied by regular breathing and the silent repetition of a Bible verse or other short phrase—can have beneficial health effects. But Benson suggests that adding strong belief to meditative prayer may trigger even more potent natural healing, perhaps through the additional release of certain chemicals in the brain and nerve cells. He cautions, by the way, that in describing these applications of belief, he does *not* rule out the possibility that healings may also occur through outside, divine intervention. He and other scientists are merely exploring the beneficial effects that strong belief may have on the body's *natural* healing processes.

As a Christian and a physician, I find such research to be quite encouraging because I do believe that there is a continuum between natural and supernatural healing. It makes sense to me that a deep faith, enhanced by a developed life of prayer and meditation, would have a positive influence on the way our God-given bodies function and heal.

On the flip side of this observation, I find that the patients with the highest levels of stress and anxiety tend to have the most physical problems. In support of my clinical observations, a Harvard School of Public Health study, reported in November 1994 in the American Heart Association's journal *Circulation,* found that men who complain of high anxiety are four to six times as likely to die from heart attacks as men who are less anxious.

A mind weighed down by cares and concerns may be the greatest threat to our health. I should know. I've always said that, over the years, I've become a "black belt" in stress management. I'm a classic Type A personality: I talk fast, take on too much work, and am tempted to become impatient when my tightly arranged schedule has to be readjusted, as it often does. In effect, I juggle five careers—practicing physician, conference speaker at about 150 functions a year, administrator of the multimillion-dollar Cooper Clinic and Aerobics Center health complex, book author, and chairman of the board and active fund-raiser for the nonprofit Cooper Institute for Aerobics Research.

Despite these self-inflicted pressures, I think that most of the time I manage the stresses in my life fairly well—for two major reasons: First, I'm able to say with the Apostle Paul, "I can do all things through Christ who strengthens me." The "Faith Factor" in my life has relieved pressures and worries as no other force I can imagine. Second, I regularly avail myself of what I've called "nature's greatest tranquilizer"—aerobic exercise. By jogging or walking at least a half hour, four or five times a week, I literally flush the tensions out of my system. A large part of this beneficial effect probably comes through the release of the neurotransmitters known as endorphins—morphine-like chemicals produced during endurance exercise.

So in my life, as well as in the lives of thousands of others whom I've treated or advised, belief and regular exercise can produce a powerful natural combination that promotes healing and well-being. If we've been given this gift, shouldn't we do all we can to take advantage of it?

QUESTION #4: AM I OPEN TO RECEIVING SPIRITUAL SUPPORT FROM OTHERS?

One of the best ways to develop an inner drive to exercise regularly is to arrange to work out with a compatible companion or a group. If you can find someone who shares your spiritual views, you'll be in a position to pursue the experience of fellowship—*koinonia,* to use the Greek term. In such a situation, the relationship with the other person or people will literally *pull* you into the exercise experience.

In one of the nation's large cities, two men, Al and Jim, were having trouble sticking to their respective exercise programs. Al, the assistant minister of an active, demanding urban congregation, was seriously overweight and sedentary. He had been told by his doctor that it was essential for him to go on a diet and start exercising, but for several reasons, the prospect of changing his habits was distasteful.

First of all, the idea of jogging or walking for a half hour or more on crowded city streets was unappealing. "If I could walk in the woods or on a beach, that would be fine," he said. "But fighting traffic and pedestrians—and smelling urine in the doorways—just doesn't motivate me."

Also, Al didn't see any way that he could rearrange his schedule to set aside the forty-five minutes to an hour in the middle of the day that was required to put on exercise gear, work out, and then shower and get dressed. He acknowledged that rising very early might be a possibility, "But I'm not a morning person," he said. "And besides, I'd feel a little nervous walking or running around on deserted streets before dawn."

The answer to Al's objections turned out to be Al's friend, Jim. Jim also needed to establish more regularity in his exercise habits, and he had wrestled with many of the same difficulties with exercise in the city that were confronting Al. Jim couldn't take time off his job as an attorney to work out in the middle of the day; he felt he was too tired to keep up a regular regimen after work; and he wasn't a "morning person" either.

But then the two men struck up a friendship during several coffee hour conversations after the church services, and they found they both enjoyed exploring deep theological and spiritual issues. Before long, they also began to discuss their mutual frustration about not being able to get started on an effective exercise program.

Finally, Al suggested that perhaps they could kill two birds with one stone: They could continue their theological discussions and, at the same time, work out together—*if* they could overcome their built-in resistance to early morning exercise. As it turned out, the mornings before work were the only time available to either of them, and so they resolved to try it. Since they lived within a few blocks of each other, they agreed that they would meet at precisely 5:30 A.M. on a certain street corner—which, by the way, had a pay phone. If one man didn't show up within five minutes of the appointed hour, the other was given permission to sound the alarm.

The arrangement worked beautifully. The two friends started their program with fast walking, graduated to a walk-jog routine, and finally were able to jog for thirty to forty minutes without stopping. As they moved along, they had the city virtually to themselves, with only an occasional vehicle or pedestrian who was heading for an early appointment. During each session together, they kept up steady conversation about religious topics, prayer techniques, and personal problems each was facing. They even prayed together while they were on the move. Their joint workout schedule lasted for nearly three years—three times a week, with breaks only for vacations and holidays.

Churchill's Foxhole Faith

Winston S. Churchill, who led Great Britain through the trials and tribulations of World War II, is often remembered as a stooped, paunchy, cigar-smoking old statesman. But in his youth, he was a fencing champion, a superb swimmer who once rescued a friend from drowning, and an expert polo player. After he graduated from Sandhurst, the British Royal Military College, he fought on the front lines on foot and horseback beside Sikhs on the Indian frontier and later was a war correspondent in the physically demanding challenges of the Boer War in South Africa.

But Churchill found at a relatively early age, when he was engaging in hand-to-hand combat against Dervish forces in India, that he needed to combine his strenuous exploits with faith. We can learn much about the need to believe in physically demanding situations from his autobiography, *My Early Life, 1874–1908*, where he writes:

I passed through a violent and aggressive anti-religious phase, which, had it lasted, might easily have made me a nuisance. My poise was restored during the next few years by frequent contact with danger. I found that whatever I might think and argue, I did not hesitate to ask for special protection when about to come under the fire of the enemy: nor to feel sincerely grateful when I got home safe to tea. I even asked for lesser things than not to be killed too soon, and nearly always in these years, and indeed throughout my life, I got what I wanted. This practice [of prayer] seemed perfectly natural, and just as strong and real as the reasoning process which contradicted it so sharply.

—from Winston S. Churchill, *My Early Life, 1874–1908* (Glasgow: Collins/Fontana Books, 1930, 1980), p. 121.

Lessons in belief and fitness from Churchill:

- Expect your faith to have practical applications.
- When physical demands increase, focus on your inner response rather than the outward challenge.

I always think back to the example set by Al and Jim when I encounter someone who says he or she lacks the motivation or opportunity to exercise. There is always a way to be motivated to begin a program, even if the solution is as simple as enlisting a close friend, a soul mate who, like you, wants to nurture the body as well as the spirit.

QUESTION #5: DO I HAVE A RELATIVELY FIRM AND STABLE PHILOSOPHY OF LIFE?

If you expect your beliefs to have a major impact in motivating you to get fit and stay fit, your deepest personal convictions must be solid and relatively unshakable. It's important to make a definite commitment about the basics of your faith and then be ready to act on that commitment. Otherwise, as James says in the Bible, you may become "double-minded" and "unstable"—characteristics of a doubting, ineffectual person who is "like a wave of the sea driven and tossed by the wind."

In my own case, as I've already indicated, I made an explicit commitment to Christ when I was still in elementary school. The only way I've found to achieve consistency in my life, including my personal fitness efforts, has been to reaffirm that commitment periodically. Yet despite the intensity and power of my own experience, I don't pretend to have a corner on the application of personal spirituality to enhance the motivation to exercise.

For example, I'm well aware that there are those who can get into shape and maintain a high level of conditioning without having any formal religious underpinning to their exercise program. But in most such cases, a strong spiritual substitute of some sort is still present. This nonreligious impetus may include a deep need to maximize one's physical potential for competition; or a medical imperative to recover from a life-threatening health crisis (such as a heart condition); or simply a desire to develop and maintain a beautiful, youthful body and energy level. Whatever the source, a strong motivating force typically emerges in disciplined exercisers, a drive that keeps them going regardless of outside pressures that may threaten to undermine discipline.

I'm reminded of one of my patients, a thirty-eight-year-old business-man named Ted, who had been a top high school athlete. He was diagnosed as having slightly elevated blood pressure, a relatively high percentage of body fat, and a low level of endurance, as indicated by a "fair" rating on a stress test he took at the Cooper clinic.

Ted was shocked at the results of his physical exam. He had not been to see a doctor since he had been checked for an insurance policy a couple of years after he had graduated from college. But he had assumed that even though he was getting a little heavier, his physical condition was still comparable to what it had been when he was a teenager. Obviously, he had been far off base—and he was startled enough to make some major changes in his life.

Believing that getting in shape was extremely important both to his health and to his self-image as an active, athletic person, Ted began to bicycle regularly—three to four days a week for thirty to forty minutes each session. Also, he embarked on a strength training program similar to the one described in chapter 8 of this book. His routine involved both calisthenics and weight workouts, three days a week. To bolster his commitment, he usually cycled with friends, who encouraged him to join them even on those days when he didn't feel quite like it.

Now, nearly ten years later, Ted has reduced his overall weight and his percentage of body fat significantly; he consistently scores in the *Superior* category for his age group on the treadmill stress test; and his blood pressure stays in the normal range without any medications. This businessman has gotten into shape and stuck with his program because of a complex of beliefs he holds about the importance of keeping fit—beliefs that have been as unwavering and stable as those of many traditional religious believers.

QUESTION #6: AM I WILLING TO STAY COMMITTED TO A PERSONAL FITNESS PROGRAM, DESPITE THE CHANGES AND NEW FINDINGS THAT REGULARLY OCCUR IN SCIENTIFIC RESEARCH?

Like your basic spiritual commitment, the commitment to a fit and healthy body should also be unwavering. But it's not always easy to remain on course, especially when a news article or TV report seems to call into question everything you have been assuming about exercise or diet.

My advice to patients who are particularly sensitive to the fickle and unstable nature of much medical journalism goes like this: When new information surfaces, you may have to make some adjustments or changes in your views about your diet or fitness program. But you must not automatically get rattled or lose heart when some new study pops up that seems to contradict what you have been taught. The news media are notorious for highlighting the most controversial elements of research, and unfortunately, these initial, often distorted news flashes are the ones that tend to become fixed in our minds.

One danger in being misled by these popular reports is the temptation to become a "health agnostic"—a skeptic who decides just to forget about fitness and diet programs because of a mistaken assumption that it's impossible to know much of anything about preventive medicine. I can still remember the initial response of some of my patients when the running guru Jim Fixx, author of the wildly popular *The Complete Book of Running* back in the late 1970s, died of a heart attack while jogging on a Vermont country road.

"I thought running was supposed to improve your health, not kill you!" one of these patients said, and some proceeded to give up their fitness programs altogether. I actually had to go on national television programs such as *Nightline* and write an entire book on the subject to set the record straight!

The Fixx fiasco was only one in a long line of distorted reports on exercise and health. About a decade later, for instance, the news media published some scientific findings indicating that cholesterol could be lowered by the soluble fiber in oatmeal. But shortly afterward, another study cast doubt on whether oatmeal could really produce this result.

"First they say one thing, and then they say another," one woman said. "I'm tempted to forget the whole fiber business and go back to my meat and potatoes."

Then there was the short-lived antioxidant controversy that arose after the publication of a 1994 study on the effects of beta-carotene supplements on middle-aged Finnish males who were heavy smokers. Contrary to a number of prior investigations, this report purportedly showed that some cancer rates went up, rather than down, after the participants took large doses of the beta-carotene. Later responses from the scientific community put the Finnish study into a more proper and limited perspective, but the fallout among some people who were influenced by the initial reports remained negative.

"Sounds to me like beta-carotene may do more harm than good," one patient told me—and it took some convincing to show him that the weight of the scientific evidence still favored beta-carotene as a preventive measure against a number of cancers.

More recently, a report suggesting that cholesterol levels aren't important in people over age seventy confused many older people who *should* continue to control their cholesterol. And you can bet that the print and electronic media will be flooded with similar unsettling reports in upcoming years.

So as you prepare to embark on a fitness and diet program, it's important to understand that there will constantly be changes, adjustments, and new findings about what you should or should not be doing in your conditioning program. But don't allow this seeming scientific uncertainty to upset or discourage you! Underneath all the flux of the new findings, there are certain constants that will remain, such as these:

- It's important to engage in regular, moderate endurance exercise.
- It's important to pursue a strength and flexibility training program throughout your life—and especially if you are middle-aged or older.
- It's important to emphasize low-fat, high-fiber foods in your diet.

From the very beginning, I've been at the center of the scientific turmoil that has gripped the popular fitness movement. When necessary, I've changed my thinking, but *without* throwing out the exercise baby with the bathwater.

A major evolution in my thinking began back in the late sixties, after the publication of my first book, *Aerobics*. At that time, I knew that the scientific evidence had established that regular exercise was essential to good health and an effective life. But I erroneously assumed that more was better—that the longer you ran, cycled, or swam, the healthier you would be.

By the time my *Aerobics Program for Total Well-Being* was published in 1982, I had shifted my thinking. In light of a deepening understanding of the role of exercise, I came to my present position that twelve to fifteen miles of jogging per week—or the equivalent other endurance exercise—is all that is required to maintain a top level of fitness and adequate protection against various diseases. Exercising more than this will significantly increase your risk of injuries. The only exception would be the person whose goal is to become a competitive athlete.

Over the years there were other important changes and adjustments that I incorporated into my thinking: During a ten- to fifteen-year period beginning in the mid-1970s, I came to see that a low-fat, low-cholesterol diet might be as important as exercise in reducing the risk of heart disease. I also became convinced about the importance of taking in relatively large quantities of antioxidants, such as vitamin C, vitamin E, and beta-carotene, to reduce the risk of heart disease, various cancers, and other illnesses. Finally, in my study of osteoporosis and the challenge of maintaining a high level of functioning as we age, I've begun to place a strong emphasis on strength programs for those over fifty. In fact, I now advocate strength training for these older groups as much as I do endurance exercise.

So there is no question that I have changed my thinking over the years—and you, too, should be ready to make necessary adjustments in your attitudes. Yet even as you retain this open, flexible perspective, it's even more important to remember the basic underlying message of *It's Better to Believe:* that your body is a temple of God, a vessel as worthy of your care as any of your most valued possessions.

How to Score Your Spiritual Checkup

To achieve the strongest possible connection between your basic beliefs about life and your fitness program—and to ensure that you'll be motivated to operate at the highest level—you should be able to answer every one of the six questions above with a yes. You'll still do well if you responded yes to five of the questions; and you can even expect progress if you give a yes to only four.

If you have positive answers on fewer than four of the questions, you may have significant trouble getting motivated to begin a regular, long-term exercise and diet transformation in your life—but don't lose heart! The great thing about a spiritual checkup is that it's always possible to improve, and in fact, *everyone* has the capacity to score 100 percent. It just may require some extra time, study, and commitment to develop this dimension of your life.

When you *do* finally begin to make some progress in strengthening your inner, spiritual fiber, you'll find that it's much easier to embark on a successful exercise regimen. And the first step that I often recommend in designing such a conditioning program is to take a close look at your body and determine precisely what is your *real* age.

4

WHAT'S YOUR *REAL* AGE?

How long—and how well—will you live?

We're told at one point by the psalmist that the normal human lifespan is seventy years, or "by reason of strength" eighty years. Earlier, in the book of Genesis, that figure is 120 years—and it's clear that many of those who lived that long, such as Abraham and Moses, weren't bedridden or incapacitated. On the contrary, they were vital and active people, who in their later years led rambunctious tribes and nations, and changed history.

In my study of the human body, I've become convinced that most of us have the innate capacity to achieve vigorous lives well up into the upper end of the biblical longevity scale, or in excess of 100 years of age. To evaluate your own potential for a long and fruitful life, it's necessary to begin with a determination of what I call your *Real Age*—the functional or physiologic age at which your physical and mental capacities are currently operating.

Of course, your Real Age and your chronological age probably won't coincide. So a man may be fifty years old chronologically, but a low level of conditioning or serious health problems may give him a Real Age of sixty. Or a woman may be fifty chronologically, but she may be in such superior shape and good health that her Real Age is only thirty-five. Obviously, it's always preferable to have a Real Age that is considerably younger than your chronological age.

Now let's turn to your situation: What do you think your Real Age is, and what does it mean in terms of what you can expect about the quality and length of your life?

How Can You Find Your Real Age?

Your Real Age depends on five main factors:

1. your current level of endurance
2. your current level of strength

3.   your current level of flexibility
4.   your current level of general health
5.   your personal and family health history

Using these five factors, you can calculate your Real Age fairly precisely, and that figure will allow you to evaluate whether you're really older or younger than your last birthday. With that information in hand, you'll be in a position to take some significant steps to "turn back the clock."

For example, the last time I calculated my Real Age, my chronological age was sixty-one years. Yet my Real Age was determined to be only forty-nine years. In other words, through a regular moderate exercise program and other measures, I actually had in a sense been able to reverse my own aging process and add on an extra twelve years of quality life. By using some simple formulas that you'll learn later in this chapter, here's what I found out about the components that make up my Real Age.

Calculating Ken Cooper's Real Age

Endurance	21 years
Strength	39 years
Flexibility	61 years
General health	60 years
Personal and family history	62 years
Total years:	243 years
Cooper's Real Age =	49 years

(243 divided by 5, rounded off to the nearest year)

Of course, a determination of your Real Age can't be made with pinpoint precision. At this time, no physician or scientist can predict exactly how long or how well you will live. But if you know where you stand with these five factors, you'll at least have a good general idea about your chances of living a long and full life. Even more important, you'll understand what changes you should make *now* to increase your potential for longevity and superior health.

Now, let's examine each of the five factors that contribute to your Real Age, and then we'll move on to some specific evaluations that will allow you to do your own calculations.

REAL AGE FACTOR #1: ENDURANCE
It's evident to me from the more than one hundred thousand people we have tested on treadmills at the Aerobics Center in Dallas that it's *not* necessary for a significant decline in endurance or aerobic capacity to occur after age forty. In fact, it seems quite possible for almost anyone who pursues

a regular endurance exercise program to maintain an extremely high level of aerobic capacity up through age forty. This means that *most* people should be capable of running, cycling, cross-country skiing, or swimming in their forties as they did in their twenties.

Of course, I'm not saying that every older person can become a world-class athlete. But I am saying there's a good chance that, with serious training, your performance as a middle-aged athlete can approach that of your earlier years, at least up to about age forty-nine. For that matter, even if you weren't in good shape in your teens or twenties, you can still get into great shape today. Many of my patients have reached their highest levels of lifetime fitness well after forty years of age.

What is the meaning of the half-century mark?   After age fifty the physical capacity of both men and women seems to decline, but not that much. Women's endurance capacities tend to decline more rapidly than men's, but I suspect that's just because older women have been more reluctant than men to plunge into regular aerobic activities. As they catch up in their interest, their times, as measured by the stress test and other procedures, will also improve.

In this regard, we've noted during the past few years that, as we recalculate our fitness classification charts every six to twelve months, the times required to achieve each level get tougher. In other words, the data we're accumulating show that more women are getting into better shape, and so we're having to rethink our standards. Furthermore, as more women become fitter with regular exercise, their age-group records edge closer and closer to the records for the men in their age groups.

What aerobic capacity should you expect as you age?   From the information we've gathered and the studies we've done at the Aerobics Center in Dallas, I'd suggest the following aerobic fitness guidelines and expectations:

- In your forties, you can approach the maximum endurance capacity you attained during your earlier years, particularly if you were never an athlete. As I mentioned earlier, if you *weren't* fit when you were younger, you can become *more* fit than you were as a youngster.
- In your fifties, you should expect some loss of endurance capacity—but not a rapid decline! A regular aerobic exercise program, of the type I'll describe shortly, will delay significantly this part of the aging process.

- In your sixties and seventies, there will continue to be a gradual decline in your endurance. But with a regular aerobic exercise program, you'll still perform better than many young people.
- In your eighties, the decline in your endurance will be more noticeable. But so long as you continue to exercise regularly—and that includes programs exclusively focusing on walking—you'll maximize your natural capacities.

What do the scientists say?   Various scientific studies on the aerobic capacities of older people support these observations about endurance that we've noted at the Aerobics Center:

- In a 1984 study in Austria, reported in the *European Heart Journal,* eight women and four men averaging over seventy-one years of age were placed on a bicycle ergometer training program. They worked about three times a week for twelve weeks at 60 percent of their maximum work capacity.

    The participants began with two ten-minute sessions for each workout and worked up to two twenty-minute sessions after six weeks. Over the course of the program, they were able to increase their maximum work load by 16 percent and their maximum oxygen uptake—a measurement of aerobic capacity—by 11 percent.
- Forty-nine veterans over age sixty-four with chronic illnesses such as arthritis, hypertension, and heart disease engaged in an exercise program over a four-month period. The regimen consisted of a warm-up, stationary cycling, stretching, weight training, walking, and a cool-down. The results: They averaged nearly a three-minute increase in their treadmill times. Furthermore, their resting heart rates decreased by an average of nearly 5 beats per minute (an indication of improved aerobic fitness).
- Various researchers—including Dr. William J. Evans (Director, Noll Laboratory for Human Performance Research at Penn State University) and exercise experts at our facilities in Dallas—have demonstrated conclusively that healthy people of *any* age can improve their aerobic capacity with regular endurance activity. Noting that physical performance is often independent of age, Evans says, "With regular exercise programs, the gains we see in VO^2 max [endurance capacity] between the old and young are similar" (*The Physician and Sportsmedicine,* Vol. 18, No. 11, November 1990, p. 89).

I'm not suggesting that exercise is a panacea which can prevent all deterioration of endurance capacity due to aging. The impact of aging is most evident among those who do little or no aerobic exercise: The heart's ability to pump efficiently will drop about 30 percent between age thirty and seventy, and the decline will continue even more precipitously after seventy.

With exercise, however, this drop in aerobic capacity can be minimized. The body's maximum pulse rate will still decline, and that means that there will be a gradual reduction in the ability to process oxygen. But regular aerobic exercise can help offset the natural decline in aerobic capacity.

You'll evaluate your own aerobic capacity with a one-mile walk test.

REAL AGE FACTOR #2: STRENGTH

Charlie, a forty-five-year-old attorney, was proud of the fact that he had kept his weight at 158 pounds, or exactly what he had weighed when he was playing intramural sports in college. He jogged a couple of miles a day, four days a week, and in general seemed in good shape for his age— that is, until he was tested for his percentage of body fat.

A measurement with calipers and underwater weighing revealed that his percent of body fat was 24 percent. That was considerably higher than he had expected and about five percentage points above what we at the Aerobics Center consider acceptable. He had not been measured for body fat when he was in college. But he was sure he hadn't been carrying that much fat in those days, and he was probably right.

In fact, as Charlie reflected on his physical condition, he realized that the shape of his body had been changing over the years. He couldn't fit into his old military uniform; the trousers were too tight around the seat, and he couldn't fasten the front button. He knew there were a couple of rolls around his middle that hadn't been there when he was twenty.

What had happened to Charlie was similar to what happens to most people as they age: He had lost muscle mass and had gained extra fatty tissue. Consequently, even though the bathroom scale gave him the same readings as twenty-five years before, his weight didn't by any means tell the whole story about his level of muscular fitness.

At the suggestion of his physician, Charlie began to include a strength training routine three times a week in his workouts. Among other things, he did exercises using light weights and included regular sets of push-ups, chin-ups, and sit-ups. Also, he lowered his daily consumption of calories by reducing his dietary fat intake from about 30 percent of his total calories to 25 percent.

As a result of these changes, when he came in for his next measurement of body fat a year later, he was a different man. His weight had gone up to 160 pounds because of his larger, better-conditioned muscles; his chest expansion increased one inch; and his waist measurement shrank by an inch. Most important, his body fat was now down to 19 percent of his total weight, or an acceptable level for good health.

The Meaning of Charlie's Transformation By increasing his muscle mass and lowering his percent of body fat, Charlie demonstrated that he was *not* too old to hold off that destructive tendency of aging, the loss of muscle tissue. Other studies suggest that you're *never* too old to reverse this aspect of aging.

Medical scientists from Tufts University have discovered that even those over ninety years of age can become stronger and increase the size of their muscles with a supervised weight-training program.

Specifically, these researchers put twelve men between the ages of sixty and seventy-two and ten men and women between the ages of eighty-six and ninety-six on a leg strengthening program. In eight weeks, the "younger" group achieved strength increases of nearly 200 percent and muscle mass increases of 15 percent. The "older" group increased their leg strength by 180 percent and their muscle mass by about 12 percent.

Without such a regular program of strength exercises—or at least consistent involvement in rigorous, muscle-conditioning activities, such as heavy labor—a steady loss of muscle mass will inevitably occur after about age thirty. By some estimates, there's a 3 to 5 percent loss of muscle mass every ten years, beginning between age thirty to forty. Some experts say that the total loss of muscle mass between ages thirty and seventy may be as high as 30 to 40 percent, or an average of 10 percent every ten years during this period. After age seventy, as most people become more sedentary, the loss of muscle mass may accelerate.

The Problem with Losing Muscle Mass What's the problem with losing muscle mass? Here are a few of the concerns:

- Less strength means a reduced ability to function physically. For example, the average 90-year-old woman must contract her thigh muscles at their maximum capacity just to stand up from a sitting position in a low chair, or to get out of a car.
- The ability to walk vigorously has been associated with longer life in older people. Specifically, a 1988 Danish study showed that gait disturbances and impairment of vision were the two objective health measurements most strongly associated with

death during a three-year follow-up among patients seventy-five to eighty-five years of age. Both aerobic exercise and strength exercises for the legs can help maintain the ability to walk efficiently.

- About 80 percent of all lower back pain results from poorly conditioned muscles. Exercise programs that strengthen the back can eliminate most of these pains after a few weeks.

The Bone Loss Link   Our bones reach a peak of density between ages twenty-five and forty. After age forty, a decline in total bone mass occurs at a rate of up to one half of one percent per year. Women who go through menopause may begin to lose their bone density at an even higher rate of 2 to 3 percent per year.

The danger in losing bone density is that there is an increased risk of broken bones and also of developing osteoporosis. This disease is characterized by brittle, porous bones that fracture easily or result in such deformities as the curved spine known as "dowager's hump." Such conditions can be debilitating and may even prove fatal. By the time they reach seventy, one-third of all women and one-sixth of all men suffer a hip fracture. Over the next five years, complications associated with these hip fractures are fatal up to 20 percent of the time.

How can you stem this tide of bone loss? It's been shown that weight-bearing exercises can help you reach the highest possible peak bone mass by age forty and then can retard the gradual loss of bone mass after age forty. Those who fail to exercise their muscles can expect to lose more bone mass than those who don't. (Treatments like estrogen replacement therapy can help overcome bone loss. For more information on this subject, see my book, *Preventing Osteoporosis,* Bantam Books, 1989.)

It's important to distinguish between the higher body weight that results from more muscles as a result of strength training, and the higher weight that comes from excess body fat. Too much body fat is associated directly with adult diabetes, high blood pressure (hypertension), high LDL ("bad") cholesterol, osteoarthritis of the lower extremities, gall bladder disease, breast cancer in women, and cancer of the colon in both men and women.

Remember, too, that you can be heavy but quite lean—or light and fat. You can see why a determination of the percent of your body fat is essential to the evaluation of your level of fitness and health.

REAL AGE FACTOR #3: FLEXIBILITY
As you age, your tendons (which connect muscles to bones) and ligaments (which connect bones to bones) begin to tighten up. The result is a loss of flexibility. But again, this aspect of aging is not written in stone. A

regular program of flexibility exercises can help keep this tendency toward stiffness at bay.

What are the benefits of flexibility? I see these main benefits to maintaining your flexibility:

- *Flexible people have a wider range of body motion and thus are able to perform movements that less flexible people find difficult or impossible.* A flexible neck enables you to look over your shoulder more easily when you're driving. Aging, in reducing this motion, can increase the difficulty and danger of looking to the rear. Overall body flexibility makes it easier to perform such common daily tasks as bending over or twisting to one side or another. Those who are more flexible are able to perform more effectively many athletic movements required in various sports.
- *Flexibility probably decreases your risk of injury.* There are different opinions on this point. But I've become convinced, after working with thousands of patients and athletes, that a regular stretching routine does help reduce the tendency to pull muscles, ligaments, or tendons, or to injure the back or joints.
- *Doing regular stretching energizes and relaxes you.* Most people's careers force them to lead sedentary lives during much of the day. Stiffness in the muscles, joints, and back may result. Aerobic and strength exercises can counter this problem, but so can stretching exercises. Working on flexibility every day—or even several times a day—is a great antidote to the stiffness and aches and pains that accompany a normal work routine.

On a personal note, as I get older I prefer to walk or jog very easily for about three hundred yards before I stretch out for a running workout. This way, I can be sure my tendons, ligaments, and muscles will be more prepared to be stretched prior to vigorous exercise. I am now recommending to my patients of all ages, but especially those over forty, that they do the same thing.

REAL AGE FACTOR #4: GENERAL HEALTH

Many times, older people who have superior endurance and also perform well on strength and flexibility tests may think they are much younger than most people of their chronological age. As a result, they may believe they really don't need to have a complete medical examination. Unfortunately, this attitude can lead to serious health problems and even early death.

A complete medical exam is as important as physical fitness. And in many cases, where there is underlying disease or illness, the exam may be *more* important. So it's essential that those over forty go in for regular physical examinations.

REAL AGE FACTOR #5: PERSONAL AND FAMILY HEALTH HISTORY

Your own personal health history and the health history of your family often exert a decisive influence on your health and fitness. For example, suppose your father or mother died of a heart attack before age fifty, or there is a history of breast cancer in your family, or you yourself have had cancer or a heart attack. In such circumstances, you're at greater risk of suffering from the same disease than those without such a history.

These areas of concern are fixed; they can't be changed. But they *can* be influenced—if you first understand where you're most vulnerable. Then, you can take steps to change those things you can change and strengthen your potential weaknesses.

Now, with this background in mind, the time has arrived to learn what your Real Age actually is.

How to Find Your Real Age

Your Real Age, then, is based on the above five components. I first referred to them when I revealed that my own Real Age was forty-nine even though I was actually sixty-one years old. These components are: endurance, strength, flexibility, general health, and personal and family history.

In order to calculate *your* Real Age, you'll have to become physically active for a few minutes so that you can take a series of simple tests. As you complete each of the physical tests or the sections of written questions, record your results on the following Real Age Master Chart. When you have filled in all the blanks, add the numbers up and divide the sum by five. That will give you your Real Age.

Real Age Master Chart

Endurance	_____ years
Strength	_____ years
Flexibility	_____ years
General health	_____ years
Personal and family history	_____ years
Total	_____ years
Real Age =	_____ years

(Add the 5 main categories and divide by 5)

But first let me offer a word of caution. If you are over forty years of age, be sure to check with your physician before taking *any* of these tests. You should also check with your physician if you're under forty and you have two or more of the following coronary risk factors: 1) Cigarette smoking; 2) high blood pressure; 3) elevated cholesterol; 4) diabetes; 5) strong family history of heart disease; 6) a personal history of being totally inactive. The presence of any of these risk factors may make it unsafe for you to take even a one-mile walking test.

TEST FOR REAL AGE FACTOR #1: ENDURANCE

To evaluate your endurance, all you have to do is take a rather simple one-mile walking test.

The One-Mile Walking Test   With this walking test, you must walk the entire distance; you can't run or jog. In other words, one foot must always be on the ground. Find a smooth, level surface where you can measure accurately a one-mile distance. Probably the easiest way to determine the mile is to use the odometer in your car. It's also fine to use a one-quarter mile track, a measured walking course in a park, or a measured course in a shopping mall.

Warm up for three to five minutes by stretching or walking briskly. Then, note the exact time on a watch with a second hand, and begin to walk—but *don't run*—for one mile as fast as you can, *without straining.* Try to move at a constant speed. On finishing the one-mile course, note the time it took you to cover the distance in minutes and seconds.

Continue to walk slowly for at least five minutes to allow your heart rate and blood pressure to return to normal. This is known as the "cool-down phase" of a workout.

To determine your endurance figure, refer to the following table. As you can see, your walking time places you in a certain age range.

For example, if you are a man and walk a mile in 11:50, your result for the endurance will be between twenty and twenty-nine years. Similarly, if you walked the mile in 13:19, your score would be between thirty and thirty-nine. For a woman, a 13:00 mile means a Real Age for this test between thirty and thirty-nine. A mile in 15:44 would be a score of fifty to fifty-nine.

To determine the specific number for your endurance score, figure the approximate fraction or percentage that your walking time has cut into the particular time category, and then apply that same fraction or percentage to the age group. For example, for men, a mile in 11:30 would equate to an age of twenty-one; 12:50 would be thirty-five. For women, 12:30 would be twenty-five; 14:45 would be forty-seven.

Endurance Test Scoring for the One-Mile Walk

Men

Real Age	Times for one-mile walking test
20–29	11:20–12:20
30–39	12:21–13:20
40–49	13:21–14:20
50–59	14:21–15:20
60–70	15:21–16:20
70+	16:21 and longer

Women

Real Age	Times for one-mile walking test
20–29	12:00–12:59
30–39	13:00–13:59
40–49	14:00–14:59
50–59	15:00–15:59
60–70	16:00–16:59
70+	17:00 and longer

Time: _____ (minutes)

Real Age for endurance: _____

(Enter this result on the Real Age Master Chart on page 44.)

TESTS FOR REAL AGE FACTOR #2: STRENGTH

After you perform the following two muscular strength tests, go directly to the short table that follows the tests. As you did in finding your endurance score, fill in the strength scores, do the calculation, and enter the final result on the Real Age Master Chart on page 44.

For example, if you are a man and can do thirty-four sit-ups in one minute, your Real Age range for sit-ups is thirty to thirty-nine years. Since your performance is at the top of that particular range, you should determine that your specific numerical score is thirty years—which is the figure you should enter on the Real Age Master Chart. If you are a woman who can do thirty-three sit-ups in one minute, you score in the range of twenty to twenty-nine years. By estimation, your specific score would be about twenty-four years—which again is the number that goes on the Real Age Master Chart.

Strength Test Part One: One Minute of Sit-ups   Lie flat on the floor on a well-padded surface, with your knees bent and feet flat on the floor. Cross your arms over your chest with hands grasping the front of each shoulder. Have someone hold your feet firmly, or slip your feet under a heavy object. Your buttocks should stay in contact with the floor at all times.

Keeping your arms or hands pressed against your body, curl your upper body off the floor to a point at which your spine is vertical or your elbows touch your knees. This movement represents one complete sit-up. *Caution:* Do not hold your breath while performing this exercise, or you may shut off the flow of blood to your head and lose consciousness.

Repeat this exercise as many times as you can in a one-minute period. Use a watch or clock with a second hand or a stopwatch so that you can determine accurately when one minute has elapsed. Enter your score and Fitness Age in the proper place below and also on the tables on page 49.

Scoring for the One-Minute Sit-up Test

Men

Real Age	Sit-ups in one minute
20–29	> 40–35
30–39	34–30
40–49	29–25
50–59	24–20
60–69	19–15
70+	< 15

Women

Real Age	Sit-ups in one minute
20–29	> 35–30
30–39	29–25
40–49	24–20
50–59	19–15
60–69	14–10
70+	< 10

Note: < means less than; > means more than.

Sit-ups _____   Real Age _____

Strength Test Part Two: One Minute of Push-ups   Standard push-ups: Place both hands on the mat or floor, approximately shoulder-width apart. The push-up test begins in the "up" position, with your arms extended perpendicular to the floor and the entire body off the floor, with only the toes and hands touching the floor.

From this up position, bend your arms and lower your body, keeping your back, buttocks, and legs in a straight line, until your chest comes within four to six inches of the floor. Do not let chest touch the floor. Push your body back to the up position, with arms extended perpendicular to the floor. This down and up movement represents one complete push-up.

The goal is to perform as many correct push-ups as you can in one minute. Use a stopwatch or clock with a second hand. Enter the results below and also in the chart on page 49.

Even though this push-up is recommended for men, women can also take this test if they desire. Likewise, men can use the modified push-ups as described below if the standard push-up is too demanding.

Modified push-ups: This push-up, designed for those who can't do the standard push-up, begins in a different kind of up position, with the knees (instead of the toes) in contact with the floor. Your lower legs should be in the air, at a forty-five degree angle with the floor. Your hands should be placed on the mat or floor, approximately shoulder-width apart, and your arms should be extended perpendicular to the floor. In this up position, all of your body will be off the floor except knees and hands.

Bend your arms and lower your body, keeping your back, buttocks, and upper legs in a straight line, until your chest comes within four to six inches of the floor. Push your body back to the up position, with arms extended perpendicular to the floor. This down and up movement represents one complete modified push-up.

The goal is to perform as many correct push-ups as you can in one minute. Use a watch or clock with a second hand.

Scoring for the One-Minute Push-up Test

Standard Push-ups

Real Age	*Push-ups in one minute*
20–29	>35–30
30–39	29–25
40–49	24–20
50–59	19–15
60–69	14–10
70+	<10

Modified Push-ups

Real Age	*Modified push-ups in one minute*
20–29	>45–40
30–39	39–35
40–49	34–30
50–59	29–25
60–69	24–15
70+	<15

Note: < means less than; > means more than.

Push-ups _____ Real Age _____

Results for Real Age Factor #2: Strength

	Score	Real Age
Sit-ups	_____	_____
Push-ups	_____	_____
Real Age for Strength =	_____	_____

(Total of both age scores divided by 2)

Now, transfer your Strength Real Age to the Real Age Master Chart on page 44.

TEST FOR REAL AGE FACTOR #3: FLEXIBILITY

The Sit-and-Reach Test   To prepare for this test, apply a piece of masking tape approximately twelve inches long to the floor. Next, place a yardstick on the floor perpendicular to the tape so that the fifteen-inch mark is flush with the front edge of the tape and the zero end of the yardstick is closest to your body. Secure the yardstick in place by putting several pieces of tape over it.

Now, you're ready for the test. With shoes off, sit on the floor. Your legs should be straight and straddling the yardstick. Keep your feet as close together as possible and your heels flush against the front edge of the masking tape. Remember, the zero end of the yardstick should be closest to your body.

With one hand on top of the other and tips of the middle fingers even, lean forward slowly with your legs straight and your arms parallel to the floor. Reach as far forward as you can over the yardstick. Be sure to keep your legs straight and don't bend your knees. Hold this position for at least one second. Do *not* bounce rapidly back and forth.

Your score is the point at which the fingertips are directly above the yardstick at the maximum reach, as documented by an observer. Your result should be recorded to the nearest ¼ inch. Perform the test three times and use the best of the three scores.

To determine your flexibility score, use the following tables. As with the other scoring tables, first determine the general Real Age range by using your performance on each test. For example, on the sit-and-reach test, a man reaching eighteen inches has a score range of twenty to twenty-nine years. Similarly, a reach of seventeen inches will give a range of fifty to fifty-nine years. Less than seventeen inches means a score of over sixty. For women, greater than nineteen inches on the sit-and-reach means a range of twenty to twenty-nine, while eighteen results in fifty to fifty-nine.

Next, to get your specific numerical score, estimate your flexibility age in five-year increments. The idea is to figure approximately where your performance places you within an age group. For example, a man who reaches halfway between 17.74 and 17.50 inches would have a specific flexibility score of thirty-five.

Scoring for the Flexibility Test
(The Sit-and-Reach Test)

Men

Real Age	Inches
20–29	18.00–17.75
30–39	17.74–17.50
40–49	17.49–17.25
50–59	17.24–17.0
60–69	16.99–16.75
70+	< 16.75

Women

Real Age	Inches
20–29	19.00–18.75
30–39	18.74–18.50
40–49	18.49–18.25
50–59	18.24–18.0
60–69	17.99–17.75
70+	< 17.75

Note: < means less than; > means more than.

Inches _____   Real Age _____

Enter the Real Age result on the Real Age Master Chart on page 44.

TESTS FOR REAL AGE FACTOR #4: GENERAL HEALTH

Physical examinations performed on a regular basis can be decisive in helping you identify life- and health-threatening diseases early. Everyone should have a complete exam at age thirty-five. A second exam should be performed at age forty and repeated every two to three years. After age fifty, complete physical exams should be done every twelve to eighteen months.

Now, here are the main elements of a general medical exam, with a few explanatory comments where they seem appropriate. As you'll see, this test has been constructed so that you always begin with your present, chronological age. Then, according to the way you answer the questions posed, you add to or subtract from that chronological age to get your Fitness Age score.

If you have had an exam within the past couple of years, you may know enough to answer the questions. Leave anything you don't know blank. After you record each of your scores here, transfer the Real Age score to the Real Age Master Chart on page 44. (When you have your next exam, you can fill in this fourth part of the test more completely.)

1. Blood Tests Have you ever been told that you are anemic or have other abnormalities in your blood?
Answers:
- No. Make no addition or subtraction.
- Yes, but no life-threatening problems. Add 2.
- Yes, and I have been told that I have a serious medical problem, such as a malignancy or leukemia. Add 10.

Score: Your chronological age _____ plus or minus additions or subtractions _____ = Real Age _____.

2. Urinalysis Do you know of any medical problems that cause your urinalysis to be abnormal?
Answers:
- No. Make no additions or subtractions.
- Yes. Add 5.

Score: Your chronological age _____ plus or minus additions or subtractions _____ = Real Age _____.

3. Blood Pressure Have you ever been told that you have high blood pressure (that is, pressures consistently above 140/90)?
Answers:
- Yes, but no blood pressure medication was prescribed. I control it with salt restriction, weight loss, or other nondrug means. Add 2.
- Yes, and I am on prescription medications. My physician says the pressure is under control. Add 3.
- Yes, and the pressure continues to be elevated, even with medications. Add 6.
- No, although the pressure is at the upper limits of normal. Make no additions or subtractions.
- No, and my physician says my readings are excellent or below normal. Subtract 5.

Score: Your chronological age _____ plus or minus additions or subtractions _____ = Real Age _____.

4. Cholesterol and Triglycerides When blood chemistry studies have been performed, have you ever been told that there are any abnormalities with your cholesterol or triglycerides?

Answers:

- No, my total cholesterol is normal. Make no additions or subtractions.
- No, my total cholesterol is very low (below 180). Subtract 5.
- Yes, my total cholesterol is high (above 200). Add 3.
- Yes, my total cholesterol is very high (above 240). Add 5.
- No, my "good" HDL cholesterol is high (above 50). Subtract 6.
- Yes, my HDL cholesterol is very low (less than 35). Add 6.
- Yes, my triglycerides are elevated (above 150). Add 3.

Score: Your chronological age _____ plus or minus additions or subtractions _____ = Real Age _____.

5. *Liver and Kidney*   Do you have any liver or kidney problems?
Answers:

- No. Make no additions or subtractions.
- Yes, but they are not life threatening. Add 2.
- Yes, I have severe liver or kidney disease which may be life threatening. Add 10.

Score: Your chronological age _____ plus or minus additions or subtractions _____ = Real Age _____.

6. *Special Laboratory Tests*   Have these revealed serious health conditions?
Answers:

- Yes, I have been diagnosed as having a positive AIDS or HIV test. Add 10.
- Yes, I have been diagnosed as having cancer from blood studies (e.g., PSA, CEA, Ca-125). Add 10.

Score: Your chronological age _____ plus or minus additions or subtractions _____ = Real Age _____.

7. *Weight*   Are you overweight?
Answers:

- Yes, but less than thirty pounds. Add 2.
- Yes, but more than thirty pounds. Add 5.
- No, I'm normal or even slightly underweight. Subtract 3.

Score: Your chronological age _____ plus or minus additions or subtractions _____ = Real Age _____.

8. *Chest Exam*   Has your physician told you that an examination of your chest was abnormal?

Answers:
- Yes, I have been told that I have lung disease. Add 5.
- Yes, I have been diagnosed as having a heart murmur or another type of heart disease. Add 5.
- Yes, my chest X ray is abnormal. Add 5.
- No, though it's been several years since I've had a chest X ray. Make no additions or subtractions.
- No, and I have a chest X ray at least every two years (if over forty years of age). Subtract 3.

Score: Your chronological age _____ plus or minus additions or subtractions _____ = Real Age _____.

9. Rectal, GI Exam   Have you had an examination of the rectum or gastrointestinal tract (the stomach and intestines) with abnormal results?
Answers:
- Yes, but the results were not life threatening. Add 2.
- Yes, and a malignancy or cancer was discovered. Add 10.
- No, and I have an annual evaluation for blood in my stool. Subtract 2.
- No, and I'm over forty and have a barium enema or colonoscopy done every five years, or a proctosigmoidoscopy done at least every two years. Subtract 5.

Score: Your chronological age _____ plus or minus additions or subtractions _____ = Real Age _____.

10. Lung Function (Spirometry)   Have you had a lung function (spirometry) test with normal results?
Answers:
- Yes, and there were no signs of obstructive or restrictive disease, including emphysema. Subtract 2.
- No, and I have been diagnosed as having obstructive disease or emphysema. Add 5.

Score: Your chronological age _____ plus or minus additions or subtractions _____ = Real Age _____.

11. ECG
   a) Have you had a resting electrocardiogram?
Answers:
- No. Make no additions or subtractions.
- Yes, and it was normal. Subtract 2.
- Yes, and it was abnormal. Add 5.
   b) Have you had a stress or exercise ECG?

Answers:
* No. Make no additions or subtractions.
* Yes, and it was normal. Subtract 6.
* Yes, and it was abnormal. Add 10.

Score: Your chronological age _____ plus or minus additions or subtractions _____ = Real Age _____.

12. PAP Test Have you had a pelvic and/or PAP test that were abnormal?
Answers:
* No. Make no additions or subtractions.
* Yes. Add 5.
* Yes, and a malignancy was discovered. Add 10.

Score: Your chronological age _____ plus or minus additions or subtractions _____ = Real Age _____.

13. Mammography Do you have mammograms performed as follows: first, for baseline results, at age thirty-five; repeated tests every two years between the ages of forty and fifty; annual tests after age fifty?
Answers:
* Yes, and the results were normal. Subtract 5.
* Yes, and the results were abnormal, but there were no signs of malignancy. Add 5.
* Yes, and a malignancy was discovered. Add 10.

Score: Your chronological age _____ plus or minus additions or subtractions _____ = Real Age _____.

14. Eyes and Vision Do you have an eye examination done regularly?
Answers:
* Yes, with no signs of glaucoma, cataracts, or other abnormalities. Make no additions or subtractions.
* Yes, and I have been diagnosed as having eye problems. Add 3.

Score: Your chronological age _____ plus or minus additions or subtractions _____ = Real Age _____.

15. Hearing Test Has your hearing been evaluated, with the result that it's normal or is adequately compensated with a hearing aid?
Answers:
* Yes. Make no additions or subtractions.
* No, I have a problem with my hearing. Add 3.

Score: Your chronological age _____ plus or minus additions or subtractions _____ = Real Age _____.

16. Dental Exam   Do you see your dentist twice a year, with the result that no major problems have been identified?
Answers:
- Yes. Make no additions or subtractions.
- No, I have a nonmalignant dental problem, such as pyorrhea, serious caries (decay), or temporal-mandibular joint syndrome. Add 2.
- No, I have oral cancer, including vocal cord cancer. Add 10.

Score: Your chronological age _____ plus or minus additions or subtractions _____ = Real Age _____.

17. Nutritional Evaluation (Fats and Cholesterol)   Do you feel that your diet is good?
Answers:
- Yes, my fat intake is less than 30 percent of my total calories, and I am consuming less than 300 milligrams of cholesterol per day. Subtract 5.
- No, my intake of cholesterol is above 300 milligrams per day. Add 5.
- No, I am consuming more than 30 percent of my calories in the form of fats each day. Add 5.

Score: Your chronological age _____ plus or minus additions or subtractions _____ = Real Age _____.

18. Alcohol   Do you have control of consumption?
Answers:
- Yes, I do not drink alcohol in any form. Subtract 5.
- Yes. I drink, but I consume fewer than ten drinks per week (a drink is 12 ounces of beer, a 1.5-ounce cocktail, or a 5-ounce glass of wine). Add 2.
- I'm not sure, but I consume more than ten drinks per week. Add 8.
- No. Add 10.

Score: Your chronological age _____ plus or minus additions or subtractions _____ = Real Age _____.

19. Drugs   Do you use drugs in any form, except those prescribed by a qualified physician?
Answers:
- No. Make no additions or subtractions.
- Yes, I do use nonprescribed, habit-forming drugs. Add 10.

Score: Your chronological age _____ plus or minus additions or subtractions _____ = Real Age _____.

This is the end of your test for General Health. Transfer all your scores in the General Health test to the following consolidated chart for General Health. By the way, don't worry too much if you have a very old Real Age score at any point in this evaluation—and don't become too ecstatic if you have one score that places you at a very young Real Age. It's the *final* Real Age calculation that really counts. We'll discuss that at the end of this chapter.

Scoring for Real Age Factor #4: General Health

Fitness Age:

1. Blood Count (CBC)   _____
2. Urinalysis   _____
3. Blood pressure   _____
4. Cholesterol and triglycerides   _____
5. Liver and kidney   _____
6. Special laboratory studies   _____
7. Overweight   _____
8. Chest exam   _____
9. Rectal, GI exam   _____
10. Lung function (spirometry)   _____
11. ECG
    a) Resting   _____
    b) Exercise   _____
12. PAP test   _____
13. Mammography   _____
14. Eyes and vision   _____
15. Hearing   _____
16. Dental exam   _____
17. Nutritional evaluation (Fats and cholesterol) _____
18. Alcohol   _____
19. Drugs   _____

Real Age Score for General Health =   _____
(Total of all ages divided by number of items tested)

Now, transfer this Real Age score to the appropriate spot on the Real Age Master Chart on page 44.

TESTS FOR REAL AGE FACTOR #5: PERSONAL AND FAMILY HEALTH HISTORY

To help you identify possible vulnerabilities in your personal or family health history, I've compiled the following list of questions, which you should ask yourself. Your responses will determine your Real Age for each subcomponent of this particular factor.

1. Personal Heart Disease   Do you have a personal history of heart disease, including coronary artery disease, congenital or inherited heart disease, heart skipping or irregularities (arrhythmias) diagnosed by a physician, a documented heart attack, balloon angioplasty, or a bypass operation?

Answers:

- Yes, but the problem occurred or was resolved over five years ago. Add 2.
- Yes, but the problem occurred less than five years ago and does not exist now. Add 4.
- Yes, the problem exists now, and I do not take medication for it. Add 10.
- Yes, and I am taking a medication for heart disease. Add 7.

Score: Your chronological age ＿＿＿＿＿＿ plus or minus additions or subtractions ＿＿＿＿＿ = Real Age ＿＿＿＿＿.

2. Family Heart Disease   Has a mother, father, brother, or sister had a history of heart disease, including coronary artery disease, angina, heart attack, bypass surgery, or balloon angioplasty?

Answers:

- No. Make no additions or subtractions.
- Yes, but the relative was over fifty years of age. Add 3.
- Yes, and the relative was under fifty years of age. Add 5.

Score: Your chronological age ＿＿＿＿＿＿ plus or minus additions or subtractions ＿＿＿＿＿ = Real Age ＿＿＿＿＿.

3. Smoking Habits   Have you ever used tobacco?

Answers:

- No, I've never used tobacco in any form. Subtract 5.
- Yes, but I quit more than two years ago. Subtract 2.
- Yes, but I quit less than two years ago. Add 1.
- Yes, I smoke only a pipe or cigar, but I don't inhale. Add 1.
- Yes, I smoke only a pipe or cigar, and I do inhale. Add 5.
- Yes, I currently smoke up to twenty cigarettes per day. Add 5.
- Yes, I currently smoke more than twenty cigarettes per day. Add 6.

Score: Your chronological age ＿＿＿＿＿＿ plus or minus additions or subtractions ＿＿＿＿＿ = Real Age ＿＿＿＿＿.

4. Diabetes—Personal   Do you have a personal history of diabetes?

Answers:

- No. Make no additions or subtractions.
- Yes, but I control it with oral medication. Add 4.
- Yes, and I require insulin. Add 7.

Score: Your chronological age _____ plus or minus additions or subtractions _____ ꞌ= Real Age _____.

5. *Diabetes—Family*　　Do you have a family history of diabetes? Answers:

- No. Make no additions or subtractions.
- Yes, my mother, father, or a sibling is an insulin-dependent diabetic. Add 3.

Score: Your chronological age _____ plus or minus additions or subtractions _____ = Real Age _____.

6. *Cancer—Personal*　　Do you have a personal history of cancer, excluding skin cancers other than malignant melanomas? Answers:

- No. Make no additions or subtractions.
- Yes, but cancer is in remission or has been cured for 5 years. Add 5.
- Yes, and cancer is still present. Add 10.
- Yes, and I'm taking radiation or chemotherapy for treatment. Add 8.

Score: Your chronological age _____ plus or minus additions or subtractions _____ = Real Age _____.

7. *Cancer—Family*　　Do you have a family history of cancer? Answers:

- No. Make no additions or subtractions.
- Yes, my mother, father, or a sibling has or has had cancer. Add 5.

Score: Your chronological age _____ plus or minus additions or subtractions _____ = Real Age _____.

8. *Chronic Diseases—Personal*　　Do you have a personal history of any chronic disease? Answers:

- No. Make no additions or subtractions.
- Yes, I have chronic kidney or liver disease (such as nephrosis, nephritis, cirrhosis, or hepatitis). Add 7.
- Yes, but my chronic disease has been cured, and there are no residual effects. Add 2.
- Yes, I have diagnosed emphysema or chronic obstructive pulmonary (lung) disease, but the problem is controlled with medications. Add 5.
- Yes, I have chronic lung disease which is still causing major, somewhat incapacitating, symptoms. Add 7.

Score: Your chronological age _____ plus or minus additions or subtractions _____ = Real Age _____.

9. Chronic Diseases—Family   Are there any chronic diseases among your family members?

Answers:

- No, there is no family history of chronic disease, including kidney or liver problems. Make no additions or subtractions.
- Yes, but the conditions are well controlled. Add 2.
- Yes, and the problems continue to exist uncontrolled. Add 3.

Score: Your chronological age _____ plus or minus additions or subtractions _____ = Real Age _____.

10. Stress   Are you having problems with stress in your life? (Note: In this context, "stress" refers to pressures associated with your job, family, or other aspects of your life.)

Answers:

- No, I am handling stress well and have no or minimal symptoms associated with stress. (Stress-related symptoms may include nervousness, anxiety, excessive worry, depression, or physical manifestations such as upset stomach or headaches.) Make no additions or subtractions.
- Yes, my stress level is moderate to heavy, but I seem to handle it well. Add 3.
- Yes, and I do not handle stress well (i.e., some of the stress-related symptoms mentioned above are present). Add 5.

Score: Your chronological age _____ plus or minus additions or subtractions _____ = Real Age _____.

Scoring for Real Age Factor #5: Personal/Family Health History

1. Personal heart disease	_____
2. Family heart disease	_____
3. Smoking habits	_____
4. Diabetes—personal	_____
5. Diabetes—family	_____
6. Cancer—personal	_____
7. Cancer—family	_____
8. Chronic disease (personal)	_____
9. Chronic disease (family)	_____
10. Stress	_____

Real Age for personal and family health history = _____
(Total of all ages divided by number of tests)

Now, transfer this final Real Age score to the Real Age Master Chart on page 44.

The Next Step

Be sure that you've transferred all the appropriate scores to the Real Age Master Chart on page 44. Do the calculation indicated there, and find your Real Age. Now, you're ready to start using this new knowledge about your Real Age, but first, let me reiterate an important point I made earlier. In determining your Real Age, my main purpose is *not* simply to try to help you predict your potential for longevity, though knowing your Real Age does give you some ideas about your chances for living a long and productive life. Rather, I mainly want to put you in a position to take action to *reverse* the aging process *by changing some of those Real Age factors that can be changed*—and as we'll see in the following pages, there are indeed many that you can improve.

Those who are more fit are less prone to die from any cause, and so I'm convinced that a well-conditioned person will be more likely to reach or exceed his or her predicted life expectancy. Perhaps even more important, a relatively young Real Age reflects an ongoing level of vigor, energy, endurance, strength, mental acuity, and emotional well-being. These are all factors that are associated with an effective, fruitful life—and can enhance your enjoyment as you serve God and others.

As I've said so many times, it's not the quantity of life that is important, but the quality. I'm inclined to agree with one of my patients who has made this statement more than once:

"I don't care so much how long I live—I just want to live *intensely* until that very last moment! I want the 'abundant life,' and I also want to be in a position where God can use me fully. Usually, I find that this means it's best for me to be healthy, relaxed, and energetic."

Next, see how *you* can begin to heighten your physical powers and emotional well-being. You'll learn to roll back the years—and achieve significant reductions in your Real Age—by improving your endurance to levels you probably never imagined were possible.

Part Two

Believing Your Way to Enhanced Endurance, Strength, and Health

5

A PROGRAM TO TAKE YOU BACK TO YOUR YOUTH

I want you to prepare to take a journey back in time—to a season or year when you can recall that you were enjoying your maximum energy and vigor. You may never have been a great athlete. In fact, you may not have been athletic at all. But just pick some bygone period when you feel you were at your physical peak—and prepare to revisit the glorious moment of your youth.

It may seem hard to believe, but by taking some relatively simple and enjoyable steps, you may actually be able to *exceed* those physical powers you possessed as a youngster! My own research and that of other exercise experts has revealed that up to about age fifty, most nonathletes who embark on a regular fitness regimen can develop levels of endurance that may be even higher than those they experienced as teenagers. Furthermore, at *any* age you can increase your muscular strength through regular strength training.

But even though you almost certainly have the potential for dramatic physical transformation, you don't have to worry about becoming some kind of fitness fanatic to achieve significant progress. Nor do you have to make abrupt or painful changes in your lifestyle. What I'm suggesting in this book is that a highly productive, active life should be a natural outgrowth or outward expression of an inner faith. When understood properly, physical fitness is something you'll *deeply desire* to achieve, and regular exercise is an activity you'll *want* to pursue—because a healthy, fit body is the most appropriate home for a vibrant spirit.

That was the discovery of a forty-two-year-old public relations consultant named Teresa, who found that she was able to move quite naturally and comfortably into a fitness program by integrating her exercise routine into her spiritual life.

Teresa's Meditation in Motion

Teresa, the mother of two, had soared to more than forty pounds above her ideal weight after the birth of her second child, and she had never been able to shed twenty of those extra pounds. The pressure of balancing her job and family life left her no free time, and so she felt she simply couldn't fit an exercise program into her schedule.

Several popular diets had worked up to a point, but she always seemed to gain back most of the weight she was able to lose. She was advised that the best way to eliminate her excess body fat was to combine a calorie-burning exercise program with a low-fat diet. But somehow, she just couldn't find the inner drive to get started on such a regimen.

Then, her life changed completely one Sunday afternoon, just after she had attended a Bible study at her church on the practice of private prayer. She was inspired to set aside fifteen minutes to a half hour every morning to have personal devotionals before the rest of the family awakened. Following this discipline was a sacrifice because Teresa cherished those extra few minutes of sleep. But she knew that progress in her spirituality depended on pursuing a prayer life, and so she was willing to make the effort. Her devotional time consisted of reading a short passage of Scripture and then spending time praying and jotting entries in a prayer journal, which her instructor had encouraged her to keep.

But this is only the beginning of Teresa's story. A couple of weeks later, her Bible instructor made a passing comment that stuck in her mind: "God doesn't demand that we sit still in one place when we pray," he said. "Some people find they fall asleep or their minds wander if they remain inactive. I know one woman who paces about her room as she prays. And there's even a man who does most of his praying as he jogs."

A light seemed to go on in Teresa's head. Suddenly she realized it just *might* be possible for her to combine her prayer life with an exercise program, and the next morning, she decided to give her idea a try. She spent the first ten minutes of her devotional time reading the Scriptures. Then she began to pray, but this time she didn't just sit in her chair. Instead, as she carried on her conversation with God, she got down on the floor and did a few stretching exercises, which she had learned long ago in a high school gym class. Finally, after about ten minutes of these flexibility movements, she returned to her chair and made her journal entries.

In the midst of this very first attempt at "meditation in motion," Teresa found that her mind was working more efficiently, and her focus on her prayer concerns was clearer. Furthermore, she had taken an all-important initial step toward a personal fitness program—and it had been not only easy, but exhilarating as well.

During the next two weeks Teresa continued her combination devotional-exercise experiment, and she even began extending the time she was spending in these sessions. At least five days a week she spent thirty, then forty, and then forty-five minutes early each morning engaging first in Bible reading, then in exercise, and finally in making her journal entries. As her program developed, she limited the Bible reading to about ten minutes, but she spent an additional five minutes memorizing verses that she found particularly meaningful.

For example, because she had been wrestling with worries and anxieties about juggling all her responsibilities, she selected the passage in Peter's first letter which advocates "casting all your care upon Him, for He cares for you." Then, repeating this short passage over and over to herself, she began her flexibility exercises. After about eight to ten minutes of stretching, she added on ten to fifteen minutes of slow walking, first just around her living room, then in her yard, and finally up and down the street in front of her home. As she moved about, she focused mainly on the verse she had memorized, meditating on its meaning and praying that God would make it a part of her daily life. In the last ten to fifteen minutes of her "meditation in motion," she returned to her favorite chair and made her journal entries.

At the end of her first three to four weeks of this activity, Teresa was feeling more energetic and alive—and she couldn't imagine returning to her previous inactive way of life. She found she was actually eager to hop out of bed in the morning and explore new physical and spiritual frontiers.

In effect, all Teresa had done up to this point was to move from a mostly sedentary person to one who engaged in a relatively low to moderate level of physical activity. But according to a study done at the Cooper Institute for Aerobics Research, which was reported in 1989 in the *Journal of the American Medical Association*, her modest effort was enough to move her into a higher health category where she faced a far lower risk of heart disease, cancer, and a variety of other life-threatening illnesses. Specifically, we found that people in the lowest 20 percent of physical activity, where Teresa had been before she started exercising, had a death rate that was 55 percent higher than those in the next 20 percent.

Just as important from Teresa's viewpoint, her increase in physical activity was making her feel more vibrant, alert, and relaxed. When combined with the devotional expressions of her faith, the exercise seemed so enjoyable and exciting that she wanted to do more. In effect, she had been working out at a level that was barely above what most experienced exercisers use for their warm-up. Even so, she was already reaping some of the most important benefits of a regular endurance program, including greater feelings of well-being and higher energy levels. And because her belief system fit so naturally into the physical activities she had chosen, she remained highly motivated to continue with her program and intensify her fitness efforts.

Teresa's experience can serve as a model for many people who are out of shape and simply can't seem to get started or maintain a regular exercise program. Your beliefs and your desire for better fitness can provide strong reinforcement for each other—*if* you want to nurture your spiritual life, and *if* you truly want to improve your physical condition.

So as you consider some of the factors that go into a solid, effective exercise and diet program, keep an open mind. Look for new, creative ways to combine your faith with your physical side. I'll periodically make some suggestions about ways to link your faith and your fitness. But in the last analysis it will be up to you to follow Teresa's lead and find your own path to spiritual and physical progress.

Getting Started

No matter what your age or current condition, it's likely that your body can reach new limits of performance. But at the outset of any conditioning program, it's essential to observe a few basic principles that will enable you to perform safely, enjoy your physical activities with a minimal risk of injuries, and reach your full physical potential. To summarize, you should:

- Get medical clearance.
- Start out slowly and progress gradually.
- Pursue all three major components of a complete conditioning program—endurance exercise, strength training, and flexibility.
- Always observe the fundamental four-step sequence for every workout: the warm-up; the main workout; the cool-down; and the strength segment.

Now here's a closer, more detailed view of these important start-up principles.

PRINCIPLE #1: GET MEDICAL CLEARANCE

You should undergo a thorough medical exam, including a stress test (an electrocardiogram under exercise conditions, such as walking on a treadmill), particularly for men over forty and women over fifty, and secure the go-ahead from a qualified physician *before* embarking on any exercise program. Tell your doctor the type of activity or sport you plan to pursue and seek his advice.

PRINCIPLE #2: START OUT SLOWLY AND PROGRESS GRADUALLY

The programs suggested in this book involve *gradual* increases in times and distances, or repetitions and resistances. Don't become impatient and jump ahead of a reasonable schedule. Take your cue from Teresa, who eased into her program—and as a result maximized her progress and enjoyment. Your body needs time to become accustomed to more demanding activity. If you try to move forward too quickly, you'll be more likely to suffer injury.

PRINCIPLE #3: ENGAGE IN ALL THREE MAJOR COMPONENTS OF A COMPLETE CONDITIONING PROGRAM

These include:

- Endurance exercise.
- Strength training.
- Flexibility workouts.

If you choose a program that has all three, you'll be prepared to age with a maximum of energy and vigor, and a minimum loss of capacity, strength, and flexibility. Programs that cover these three types of exercise are described in the following chapters.

PRINCIPLE #4: ALWAYS OBSERVE THE FOLLOWING FOUR-STEP SEQUENCE FOR A WISE WORKOUT

Step One: Warm up.   Many pulled muscles result from a failure to ease into the main part of the workout. This "easing in" is the function of the warm-up, which should last a minimum of three to five minutes.

One of the best ways to warm up is to perform the movements that mimic the primary exercise you plan to do, but at a less intense pace. For example, if you're a walker, you might try walking at about three-fourths the speed of your regular workout as a warm-up. This way, your muscles, ligaments, and tendons will be stretched and prepared for the more demanding work that is to come later.

Another way to warm up is to do *light* strength-oriented calisthenics (or weight work, if you're about to begin a weight-training session). But I want to emphasize the word "light." If you work too hard during the warm-up phase, you may become overly fatigued by building up what we call an oxygen debt. In simple terms, you'll become winded or *anaerobic,* and feel much the way you would after doing a series of sprints. This excessive demand on the body at the very beginning of the workout can also lead to injuries or other health problems.

Finally, you can warm up by doing very slow, light stretching exercises. Again, I want to emphasize the easy nature of these movements.

There's been a mistaken assumption that the warm-up should consist of vigorous stretching from the outset. This misconception arises from a failure to recognize that it's actually necessary to warm up *before doing demanding flexibility movements,* as well as before other types of exercise! If you don't warm up before trying a strenuous stretch, you increase the chances that you'll pull a muscle, ligament, or tendon.

Step Two: Do the main part of your workout.   This will involve your primary endurance activity, if that is on your schedule. Or it may involve your main strength or flexibility work. Examples of these programs are included in later chapters.

Step Three: Cool down.   Take at least five minutes after the main part of your workout to walk about slowly, swing your arms around, or otherwise move at a lessened pace. This way, you'll allow your body to return gradually to a resting state. Those who fail to follow this third step and abruptly stop all activity may experience extreme discomfort until their heart rate has returned to normal. Even more serious cardiac (heart) abnormalities may occur when the exerciser stops too suddenly. Remember, a higher percentage of severe heart problems occur within five minutes after exercise, not during the main part of the workout.

Step Four: If you plan to do all your exercises on the same day, schedule your main strength exercises after the endurance phase of the workout.   Although many people like to combine their endurance and strength work, it's important to position any strength exercises after the cool-down phase of the endurance program. Otherwise, you'll be likely to build up the oxygen debt I mentioned in Step One.

Of course, you can always do your strength training on different days from those you devote to aerobic exercise. In that case, you won't have to worry about when you should perform this exercise, though you'll still have to go through the usual warm-up and cool-down procedures.

These are the general principles you should keep in mind for each of the three main exercise objectives—flexibility, endurance, and strength. Now, let's move on to the specific programs, which have been designed to keep you vigorous, energetic, strong, and physically fit for the rest of your life.

Make Use of Your Memory

In his *Confessions,* St. Augustine waxed eloquent on the wonder and power of memory:

> *In my memory are sky and earth and sea, ready at hand along with all the things that I have ever been able to perceive in them and have not forgotten. And in my memory too I meet myself—I recall myself, what I have done, when and where and in what state of mind I was when I did it. In my memory are all the things I remember to have experienced myself or to have been told by others. . . . I can picture actions and events and hopes for the future; and upon them all I can meditate as if they were present. . . . Great is this power of memory, exceedingly great, O my God, a spreading limitless room within me. Who can reach its uttermost depth? Yet it is a faculty of my soul and belongs to my nature. In fact, I cannot totally grasp all that I am.*
>
> —trans. by F.J. Sheed from *The Confessions of Saint Augustine, Books I–X* (New York: Sheed & Ward, 1942), pp. 179–180.

Lessons on the use of memory from St. Augustine:

- In planning your exercise sessions, always include a spiritual dimension that makes use of your memory. For example, you might memorize a short passage from Scripture or from a favorite book, and then turn the words over in your mind as you work out. Contemplate their meaning, as you walk, run, or cycle.
- If you are confronting a particularly difficult problem at work or home, frame the issue clearly before you exercise—and then "hold" the idea or problem in your mind. Don't try to wrestle or struggle with it. Instead, let your thoughts drift back and forth to your concern as you exercise. Most likely, as you allow your memory and thinking processes to develop a life of their own in this way, a creative solution will come to mind in some way you have never expected.

6

STRETCHING YOUR BODY AND SPIRIT

Light flexibility exercises are often placed at the beginning of a workout to give the body a chance to warm up, and along with the increased circulation and muscle readiness comes a sense that you have, quite literally, *stretched* your body's potential to a new plane of suppleness and range of motion.

When you do a proper stretch, you gently push and pull your muscles, ligaments, and joints slightly beyond the point of comfort. You don't jerk your body about, and you certainly don't push to the point of pain, because that could easily cause injury. But unless you move a little past your normal comfort zone, you'll never experience any progress.

The physical experience of stretching can serve as a kind of metaphor when an opportunity for spiritual growth arises. We're told in the New Testament book of Acts, for instance, that after Peter preached at Pentecost and three thousand new believers made decisions to follow Christ, the new converts devoted themselves to four pursuits: prayer, the breaking of the bread (probably the Lord's Supper), fellowship, and the Apostles' teaching (the equivalent of Bible study for us today). Just as stretching the spirit through effort and discipline is required to achieve spiritual progress, physical improvement also depends on increasing the flexibility of various parts of the body.

What Kind of Stretching Is Important

Good flexibility helps minimize injuries and maximize athletic performance. The wider your range of motion, the more efficiency, speed, and power you can achieve. This means it's important to work on flexibility in all the major parts of your body. Specifically, you should stretch each of these muscle groups at least three times a week:

- rear shoulders and upper back
- back of the upper arms, and middle and sides of the back
- hamstrings (back of thighs) and lower back

- groin
- lower back and buttocks

As time permits, you may want to add other flexibility exercises, over and above the ones I'm suggesting. But regardless of what flexibility program you choose, you should keep in mind these basic principles for safe stretching:

- All movements should be done slowly, without any bouncing or fast motion.
- Work on achieving a full range of motion.
- Work up gradually to your full stretching ability. It may take half of a stretching workout to achieve this target.
- At some point in the workout, hold your maximum stretch on each exercise for about fifteen seconds; then slowly relax your body as you return to the starting position.

These exercises should take only about ten minutes to complete and may be performed at various points in an exercise program. For example, they might be included in the warm-up, in the cool-down, or as part of the strength workout.

The Fundamental Flexibility Program

THE FLAT-ON-YOUR-BACK STRETCH

Lie flat on your back, and extend your arms over your head on the floor. Point your toes and stretch your arms as far as possible beyond your head. Hold the stretch for five seconds. Relax and repeat three times.

This stretch will help you "unwind" the muscles along the entire length of your arms, trunk, and legs.

LEG EXTENDER

Lie on your back, with legs extended straight out on the floor, and thighs and feet touching. Extend your arms on the floor straight out from your shoulders and perpendicular to your body.

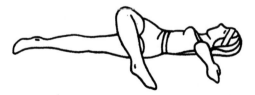

To begin the exercise, move your right leg up and over your left leg, and place it on the floor as close as possible to your extended left hand. To achieve this position, you'll make a twisting movement with your hips and lower body. Return to the starting position. Keep your shoulders firmly on the ground throughout. Repeat the movement three times with each leg.

This stretch will enhance the flexibility of your hips, hamstrings, and lower back.

MacArthur's Muscular Prayer

General Douglas MacArthur, the great commander of Allied forces in the Pacific during World War II, began every morning with a round of calisthenics, walked miles every day, avoided alcohol, and saw regular exercise as essential to the whole person. He liked to quote the philosopher John Dewey: "There is an impossibility of insuring general intelligence through a system which does not use the body to reach the mind and the mind to teach the body."

MacArthur's religion was unorthodox. Though he believed in God, he placed a heavy emphasis on evangelizing through foreign missionaries to promote the "democratic concept." Still, his beliefs seemed to help him put his independent, self-reliant nature into a broader spiritual perspective. Consider, for instance, this portion of a prayer he wrote after supper one evening for his young son, Arthur:

Build me a son, O Lord, who will be strong enough to know when he is weak, and brave enough to face himself when he is afraid; one who will be proud and unbending in honest defeat, and humble and gentle in victory.

Build me a son whose wishes will not take the place of deeds; a son who will know Thee—and that to know himself is the foundation stone of knowledge.

Lead him I pray, not in the path of ease and comfort, but under the stress and spur of difficulties and challenge. Here let him learn to stand up in the storm; here let him learn compassion for those who fail.

—from William Manchester, *American Caesar: Douglas MacArthur, 1880–1964* (Boston: Little, Brown and Company, 1978). pp. 123, 164–165, 314, 511–512.

Lessons in belief and fitness from MacArthur:

- Regular exercise is necessary to maximize your mental powers—and the morning is often the best time for a workout.
- The pursuit of flexibility and strength should always occur in a spiritual framework.

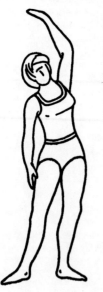

SIDE STRETCHER

Stand up straight, with your right arm relaxed at your side and your left arm extended above your head. Your feet should be approximately three feet apart.

Bend your trunk to the right, keeping your left arm extended above your head. Return to the starting position. Your feet should remain on the floor. Repeat this movement with your right arm extended and your body bent to the left side. These movements, both to the right and to the left, constitute one repetition. Perform a total of ten repetitions.

This stretch will add flexibility to your waist and the sides of your back.

BACK-OF-THE-ARM AND SIDE-OF-THE-BACK STRETCH

You may begin in a standing or sitting position. Lift your right elbow toward the ceiling, and place your right hand as far down on your back as possible between the shoulder blades. This is similar to what you would do with a "scratch your back" movement. Allow your chin to relax on your chest.

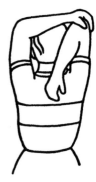

Your left hand should then gently pull your right elbow to the left until a stretch is felt on the back of your right arm and down the right side of your back. Hold this position for fifteen seconds. Repeat the movement once with your left elbow and arm being pulled down by your right hand.

This exercise stretches the triceps muscles, which are found on the back of the upper arm, and the latissimus dorsi muscles, which extend across the middle and lower back.

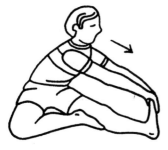

HAMSTRING AND LOWER BACK STRETCH

Sit with your left leg extended in front of you. Your left foot should be flexed, with the toes pointing toward your upper body and your left kneecap facing the ceiling. Your right knee should be bent and your right foot placed flat against the side of your left knee.

Without rounding the back, lean forward from the hip over your left leg. Extend your hands toward your left toe, with eyes looking straight ahead. When you feel a tightness behind your left leg, hold the position for fifteen seconds.

Then, move to the second part of the exercise, which stretches the lower back. Bend forward toward your left foot by "rounding" your back forward over your left leg. Try to bring your nose as close as possible to your left knee. When you've stretched as far as you comfortably can toward the knee, hold the position for about fifteen seconds.

Repeat both these stretches with your right leg.

REAR ANKLE RAISE

From a standing position, reach behind your back and grasp your left foot with your right hand. You may want to steady your balance by placing your left hand against a wall or railing. Then, using your right hand, slowly pull your left foot toward your buttocks. You should feel your left thigh muscle stretching. When you feel a good, comfortable stretching sensation on the front of your left leg, hold this position for fifteen seconds. Repeat two times with each leg.

Note: If you have trouble doing this exercise while standing, it's just as effective to perform the stretch while lying on your side or stomach.

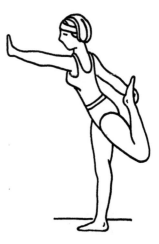

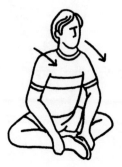

GROIN STRETCH

Sit on the floor with the soles of your feet together. Hold your legs just above the ankle, and place your elbows on your inner thigh, close to your knees. Slowly, pull your feet as close to your body as possible. Then, gently press your thighs open and down with your hands. You'll feel a stretching sensation in the upper, inside part of your thighs and your groin. When you reach the greatest tension that you can manage with this stretch, hold for fifteen seconds.

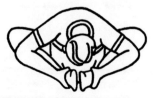

LOWER BACK STRETCH

Lie flat on your back on the floor, with your legs together and extended against the floor, and your arms resting comfortably on the floor out from your sides.

Raise your right knee up toward your chest, grasp your knee with both your hands, and pull your knee as close to your chest as you can. You should feel your lower back stretching out, and you may even hear a few segments of your spine pop! Hold this position for fifteen seconds.

Repeat this motion with your left knee.

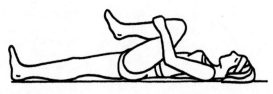

Next, raise *both* your knees up toward your chest, grasp them with your hands, and pull them as close to your chest as possible. Hold for fifteen seconds.

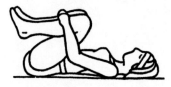

Finally, while still lying on your back, flex your legs so that your knees are off the floor and the soles of your feet are flat on the floor. Flatten your spine against the floor so that the normal curve of your lower back is pressed against the floor. Hold for fifteen seconds.

This exercise is considered one of the best for stretching out the lower back and helping to prevent pulls or muscle injuries to the lower back.

ACHILLES TENDON STRETCH

Stand about two or three feet from a wall or railing, with your right foot about eighteen inches to two feet in front of your left, as though you were in the process of taking a step or stride. The heels of both feet should be touching the floor. Lean over so that you are supporting your weight against the wall or railing with your hands. Push against the wall so that you feel an increasing tension in the back part of your lower legs and the back of your ankles, where the Achilles tendon is located. Hold this position for fifteen seconds, and then repeat with your feet in the reverse position.

If you do these exercises at least three times a week, you'll begin to see real progress in your flexibility. Also, because they are performed in a slow, quiet, and deliberate fashion, they can be combined quite effectively with spiritual practices, such as prayer, meditation, Bible memory work, or simply the often-overlooked discipline of silence.

In any event, no matter how you choose to work a flexibility routine into your daily life, these stretches will constitute a great warm-up for the other parts of your fitness program such as the endurance exercises we are now going to discuss.

7

THE SECRET TO GREATER ENERGY AND STAYING POWER

Whenever I read the words of Isaiah that say those who "wait on the LORD" shall "run and not be weary" and "walk and not faint," I'm reminded of how naturally spiritual development and endurance exercise go together. As the prophet suggests, inner staying power can enhance physical staying power.

How exactly does this interaction work? Much of our wasted energy, including our tendency to feel fatigued early in the day or to "run out of steam" before a task is complete, arises from an inability to handle stress well. I can't count the number of times I've heard patients who are under severe personal, family, or career stress complain that they are always tired or have lost interest in life. Others focus on the fact that they are constantly distracted and generally inefficient in their work or volunteer efforts because of "too many things on my mind." Yet when the source of stress is removed from these very same patients, their energy, vitality, and efficiency return.

Endurance exercise by itself can be a great stress reducer and source of relaxation. But it has also been my experience that a physical program works best when it's accompanied by a tranquil mind and spirit.

I'm reminded of the complaint of one patient (a complaint, I might add, that I've voiced myself) that "I really can't enjoy a workout fully when I have too many things on my mind." He observed that, up to a point, endurance exercise could overcome the cares of the day. But when the cares and concerns were too great, and the related anxieties overwhelming, the physical workout helped little, if at all.

His antidote to very high levels of stress was first to attend to his spiritual needs. Sometimes, he would find a solitary place, and, in his imagination, he would "cast all his cares" on God, as Peter suggests. Other times, he might go through the prayer sequence Paul outlines in the fourth chapter of his letter to the Philippians, with first a supplication to overcome anxiety, and then a time of giving thanks for his blessings. When this man had spent even a few minutes in this sort of meditative prayer, he usually found he was better prepared to enjoy his physical workout to the fullest.

What all this suggests is that if things are generally right in your inner being *before* you work out, the benefits of your aerobic fitness program will most likely be magnified. Of course, because we don't live in a perfect world, you can't expect your inner house to be entirely in order every time you go out for a walk, jog, or swim. But to realize the maximum potential of your physical activity, I do recommend that, whenever possible, you try to spend some time focusing on the spiritual dimension of your life *before* you attempt to engage in your regular endurance exercise routine. By dedicating even a few moments to such focused thinking or prayer, you can establish a kind of spiritual momentum which will carry over to your entire workout.

I've known many people who begin the day with a Bible reading and prayer, and then they'll go out for their walk or jog. Others may start things off by reading some philosophical or inspirational literature. The idea is to choose a quiet activity that will stimulate your inner life and prepare you to continue your reflections when you become more active.

What kinds of activities will increase your physical endurance and at the same time serve as a natural extension of your spiritual side? To help you answer this question, I'll first provide a brief overview of the possibilities, and then we'll explore in more detail each of the major endurance programs.

Specific Programs to Enhance Your Staying Power

The specific endurance programs in this chapter include systematic, graduated exercises for a variety of activities. These programs are designed to improve your aerobic and cardiovascular capacity and should be the cornerstone of your fitness efforts. As an added benefit, a meditative state of mind may be encouraged by the repetitive nature of these activities. Also, properly performed, endurance exercises shouldn't result in the mental distraction that arises from physical exhaustion. This is because they are designed to be performed at only about two-thirds to three-fourths of your maximum exercise capacity or heart rate. Now here are some of the possible activities you can choose:

- walking
- treadmill walking
- running/jogging
- outdoor cycling
- stationary cycling

- swimming
- miscellaneous endurance programs, such as:
    - aerobic dancing
    - stair climbing
    - stationary running
    - rope skipping
    - step aerobics
    - rowing machines
    - cross-country ski simulators

Although the main purpose of these exercises is to improve your endurance, they will also strengthen specific muscles related to the sport or activity involved.

The general principles of exercise described in the previous two chapters still apply. So be sure that you include a medical checkup, a warm-up, and a cool-down, which are all necessary to a successful and safe workout. Now, it's time for you to select an endurance program.

How to Select a Personal Endurance Program

First, pick one of the following activities and follow the instructions accompanying the exercise.

Second, start out with the graduated, age-related Beginner's chart for the program you've selected. Don't try a work level that is too demanding, or you could hurt yourself. You have plenty of time to get into shape, so enjoy it! Also, the less you are forced to focus on sore muscles or a fatigued body, the more opportunity you'll have to consider creative ways to incorporate the practices of faith, such as prayer and meditation, into your workout.

Third, when you reach the top level of conditioning for the Beginner segment of the program for your age group, consider moving on to the Recreational level—but only if you think you'd like more of a physical challenge. If you're content exercising in the Beginner range, you'll still receive plenty of benefits for your health and well-being.

Fourth, if you get into good shape on the Recreational program and want to move on to an even more demanding activity, you might try the Elite level, which is most appropriate for those interested in competitive endurance events. But again, take this step only if you feel you'd enjoy the challenge.

Note: So long as you increase your conditioning gradually and systematically, you'll still be operating safely, even at the Elite level. In other words, your risk of muscular and skeletal injuries will be minimal. Furthermore, as I mentioned in my book, *Antioxidant Revolution,* the rigor of

A pair of tourists entered the Church of St. Peter on the shores of the Sea of Galilee and made a surprising discovery:

We had the church and shore to ourselves, except for a solitary supplicant wearing a long dark brown habit with rope sash. He was huddled in a corner in an attitude of prayer, and so we walked quietly about the interior of the small stone chapel in an effort not to disturb him. We were about to go outside again and sit on some rocks on the lakeshore when I saw the man swat at a couple of flies that were swarming about his head. Since his concentration in prayer had apparently been broken, I decided to approach him on the chance that he might speak English.

Not only did he speak English, but he spoke it with an Ohio accent, and he was eager to talk. He introduced himself as Father Arcadius, a Franciscan priest from Cleveland, and explained that he had spent more than a year, mostly on foot, trekking from Italy to Israel. He planned to spend a considerable amount of time wandering up and down the hills of the Holy Land—again, on foot. Here was a man engaging in true first-century exercise!

But his goal was obviously not primarily the improvement of his cardiovascular system. "I just want to adore God, be with Jesus, because he was rejected by so many," he told us. "And I pray best when I'm walking at a steady pace."
—from William Proctor, "Running Where Jesus Walked," *Christian Herald*, April 1979, p. 32.

Lessons from Father Arcadius, the "walking priest":

- The steady rhythm of aerobic walking—which is fast enough to get a cardiovascular benefit, but not so exhausting as to interfere with creative thought—is an ideal medium to pursue private prayer.
- Consistency is more likely when regular exercise is done in accordance with an overriding spiritual purpose.

exercise will not be so extreme as to produce excess "free radicals," or unstable oxygen molecules in the bloodstream, which could increase your risk of various diseases.

Finally, when you're participating in endurance exercise, you'll experience the greatest fitness benefits if you monitor how you *feel* about the effort you're putting out. When you first begin, a program should involve at least "fairly light" effort, and then in later weeks you should move on to a "somewhat hard" to "hard" degree of intensity.

This may seem a rather vague way to evaluate how much effort you're exerting. But actually, a scientifically tested scale known as the "Borg Rating of Perceived Exertion" has shown this subjective approach to work quite well. After they move beyond the first couple of weeks of a program, most exercisers who feel that they are working out somewhere in the range of "somewhat hard, but still feels fine," to "hard and heavy," will get all the endurance benefits they need. But if you feel you're working "very hard," you've gone too far—unless you're striving for a competitive level of training.

Now, with these guidelines in mind, select one of the following endurance programs.

The Endurance Programs

THE WALKING WORKOUT

What are the real benefits of walking?   In the past, walking has sometimes been the "poor cousin" to other aerobic activities. I've always included walking as one of the five top aerobic activities—along with jogging, cycling, swimming, and cross-country skiing. But those of us in the fitness and preventive medicine fields have often recommended walking to people who weren't able to jog or run, as the initial step that would lead eventually to jogging or running.

But now we are learning that walking is an excellent exercise in itself. A comprehensive investigation on walking was conducted at our Institute for Aerobics Research in Dallas, with the report published in the December 18, 1991, issue of the *Journal of the American Medical Association.*

Under the leadership of Dr. John Duncan, our research staff performed a six-month study involving 102 premenopausal, healthy women. One group of women acted as a control group, without any significant changes being made in their exercise habits. The three other groups trained at different walking speeds. The first groups walked twenty minutes per mile; a second group walked fifteen minutes per mile. After a few weeks of specialized training, a third group was able to walk twelve minutes per mile.

Each of the three exercising groups walked three miles per day, five days per week for a six-month period. They covered more than 20,000 miles during that time, and not a single injury requiring a physician's care occurred—a clear testimony to the safety of walking.

After six months, improvement in aerobic fitness was documented in each of the exercising groups by showing an increase in the "maximal oxygen consumption," the standard test for cardiovascular fitness. The group walking twenty minutes per mile increased their aerobic fitness by 4 percent. The fifteen-minute-per-mile group increased their fitness by 9 percent. And the twelve-minute milers improved their aerobic fitness by 14 percent.

In other words, the aerobic benefit was dose-related. The faster the speed, the greater the response. (Because of the technique and muscle groups used, very fast walking can actually be more beneficial aerobically than jogging or slow running at the same speed.)

Findings on the participants' heart rates during exercise are also of interest. The twenty-minute milers exercised at an average of only 56 percent of their predicted maximal heart rate. The fifteen-minute-milers worked out at 65 percent of their predicted rate. And the twelve-minute milers moved along at an amazing 86 percent of their predicted maximal heart rates. The twelve-minute per mile walkers expended as much energy and reached the same heart rates as those women who ran nine-minute miles! Walking that fast takes a lot of energy. If you don't believe me, try it!

There were also other health benefits among the walkers in this study. The most significant change was noted in their HDL, or "good" cholesterol. The twenty-minute milers had a 6 percent increase—the same as the twelve-minute milers! Studies indicate that for every one percent you can increase the HDL cholesterol, you decrease the incidence of coronary heart disease by 3 percent. Therefore, both the twenty-minute walkers and the twelve-minute walkers decreased their risk of heart disease by 18 percent!

Walking is obviously quite effective both in improving aerobic fitness and also in improving health. I believe this so firmly that I've inserted walking sessions into many of my weekly endurance routines. So it's with good reason that this activity leads off our endurance program selections.

GUIDE TO THE WALKING PROGRAMS

1. To keep track of your distances, measure a flat, straight, curved, or rectangular surface equal to the mileage you expect to walk.

2. After a three-minute warm-up of calisthenics or moderate-paced walking, walk the prescribed distance at the beginning of the week, but don't worry too much about your speed. By the end of the week, attempt to reach the stated time goal. Arms should be swinging freely throughout the workout. If you can't achieve the final goal, repeat the week.

3. Always cool down with slow walking for five minutes after completing the measured distance.

4. In the Beginner program, it's assumed that the exerciser has no previous aerobic conditioning.

5. The Recreational program has been structured for the walker who is already involved in a regular program and wants to improve his or her speed.

6. The Elite program is designed for the competitive aerobic walker, or the race walker. If a faster speed is desired and there are no medical restrictions, you can follow one of the programs for younger people.

7. The handweight option is only for the last four weeks of the Beginner program. Adding the handweights will decrease both the required dura tion of the activity and the number of times per week that it's necessary to work out to achieve an adequate training effect.

For aerobic (Recreational) and race (Elite) walkers, it's recommended that handweights not be used. Handweights also shouldn't be used by those seventy and older. At faster walking speeds, or when relatively old bodies are involved, handweights may cause musculoskeletal injuries to the arms and shoulders.

8. By the final week of each program, an adequate level of aerobic conditioning will be reached. This level can be maintained on a schedule that involves four to five sessions per week. If you've reached the top level

of the Beginner program and want to move on to the Recreational program, or if you've reached the top level in the Recreational Program and want to try the Elite program, begin the next program at the lowest level indicated by the appropriate chart.

9. An "x" in front of a number in parentheses in the Elite program refers to an interval training workout, a concept that involves covering relatively short distances in very fast times. Interval workouts are helpful in increasing race times.

In week four of the up-to-forty-nine-years Elite program, for instance, the exerciser should first walk three miles in thirty-six minutes. Then he should walk two one-mile distances (indicated by "x2"), at a pace of 11:30 per mile, with a two-minute rest in between, as noted on the chart.

10. All the programs can be used by men or women.

11. It's essential for every exerciser to secure medical clearance, including a stress electrocardiogram, before beginning a Recreational or Elite walking program.

Walking Exercise Programs (To 49 years)
Beginner
Goal: 14:30/mile pace

Week	Distance (miles)	Time Goal (minutes)	Frequency/Week (sessions)
1	2.0	36:00	3–5
2	2.0	35:00	3–5
3	2.0	34:00	3–5
4	2.0	33:00	3–5
5	2.5	42:00	3–5
6	2.5	40:00	3–5
7	2.5	38:00	3–5
8	3.0	47:00	3–5
9	3.0	45:00	3–5
10	3.0	<43:00	3–5

Handweight Option for Last Four Weeks

(three-pound weight in each hand, actively swinging the arms)

7	2.0	32:00	4
8	2.0	30:00	4
9	2.5	38:00	4
10	2.5	<37:00	4

< means less than

Recreational
Goal: 13:30/mile pace

Week	Distance (miles)	Time Goal (minutes)	Frequency/Week (sessions)
1	2.0	30:00	3–5
2	2.0	28:00	3–5
3	2.0	27:30	3–5
4	2.5	35:00	3–5
5	2.5	34:30	3–5
6	2.5	34:00	3–5
7	3.0	42:00	3–5
8	3.0	41:30	3–5
9	3.0	41:00	3–5
10	3.0	<40:30	3–5

< means less than

Elite (Race Walkers)
Goal: 11:30/mile pace

Week	Distance (miles)	Time Goal (minutes)	Frequency/Week (sessions)
1	3.0	36:00	5–6
2	4.0	50:00	5–6
3	5.0	62:00	5–6
4	3.0	36:00	3
	1.0 (x2)	11:30 2:00 rest	3
5	3.0	35:00	4
	0.5 (x4)	5:30 1:30 rest	2
6	4.0	48:00	4
	0.25 (x8)	2:30 1:00 rest	2
7	3.0	35:00	3
	2.0	24:00	3
8	5.0	58:00	2
	1.0 (x3)	10:45 2:00 rest	4
9	4.0	46:00	3
	0.5 (x4)	5:15 1:00 rest	2
10	3.0	<33:00	5

< means less than

Walking Exercise Programs (50–59 years)
Beginner
Goal: 15:00/mile pace

Week	Distance (miles)	Time Goal (minutes)	Frequency/Week (sessions)
1	1.5	30:00	3–5
2	1.5	28:00	3–5
3	2.0	38:00	3–5
4	2.0	36:00	3–5
5	2.0	34:00	3–5
6	2.5	42:00	3–5
7	2.5	40:00	3–5
8	2.5	38:00	3–5
9	3.0	47:00	3–5
10	3.0	46:30	3–5
11	3.0	45:00	4
12	3.0	<45:00	4

Handweight Option for Last Four Weeks
(three-pound weight in each hand, actively swinging the arms)

Week	Distance (miles)	Time Goal (minutes)	Frequency/Week (sessions)
9	2.0	32:00	4
10	2.0	30:00	4
11	2.5	39:00	4
12	2.5	38:00	4

< means less than

Recreational
Goal: 14:00/mile pace

Week	Distance (miles)	Time Goal (minutes)	Frequency/Week (sessions)
1	2.0	32:00	3–5
2	2.0	30:00	3–5
3	2.0	28:00	3–5
4	2.5	36:00	3–5
5	2.5	35:00	3–5
6	2.5	34:30	3–5
7	3.0	43:00	3–5
8	3.0	42:30	3–5
9	3.0	42:00	3–5
10	3.0	<42:00	3–5

< means less than

Elite (Race Walkers)
Goal: 11:30/mile pace

Week	Distance (miles)	Time Goal (minutes)	Frequency/Week (sessions)
1	3.0	39:00	4–5
2	3.5	45:30	4–5
3	4.0	52:00	4–5
4	3.0	38:00	3
	1.0 (x2)	12:30 2:00 rest	3
5	3.0	37:00	4
	0.5 (x4)	6:00 1:30 rest	2
6	4.0	50:00	4
	0.25 (x8)	2:45 1:00 rest	2
7	3.0	36:00	3
	2.0	24:30	3
8	4.0	48:00	2
	1.0 (x3)	11:00 2:00 rest	4
9	4.0	46:00	3
	0.5 (x4)	5:30 1:30 rest	2
10	3.0	<34:30	4–5

< means less than

Walking Exercise Programs (60–69 years)
Beginner
Goal: 17:00/mile pace

Week	Distance (miles)	Time Goal (minutes)	Frequency/Week (sessions)
1	1.0	24:00	3–5
2	1.0	22:00	3–5
3	1.0	20:00	3–5
4	1.5	32:00	3–5
5	1.5	31:00	3–5
6	1.5	30:00	3–5
7	2.0	40:00	3–5
8	2.0	39:00	3–5
9	2.0	38:00	3–5
10	2.5	47:00	3–5
11	2.5	45:00	4
12	2.5	42:30	4

Handweight Option for Last Four Weeks
(three-pound weight in each hand, actively swinging the arms)

9	1.5	32:00	4
10	1.5	30:00	4
11	2.0	40:00	4
12	2.0	39:00	4

Recreational
Goal: 15:00/mile pace

Week	Distance (miles)	Time Goal (minutes)	Frequency/Week (sessions)
1	1.5	27:00	3–5
2	1.5	25:00	3–5
3	1.5	24:00	3–5
4	2.0	32:30	3–5
5	2.0	31:45	3–5
6	2.0	31:00	3–5
7	2.5	39:00	3–5
8	2.5	38:00	3–5
9	3.0	47:00	3–5
10	3.0	< 45:00	3–5

< means less than

Elite (Race Walkers)
Goal: 13:00/mile pace

Week	Distance (miles)	Time Goal (minutes)	Frequency/Week (sessions)
1	2.0	30:00	4–5
2	2.5	37:30	4–5
3	3.0	45:00	4–5
4	4.0	60:00	4–5
5	3.0	44:00	3
	1.0 (x3)	14:00 2:00 rest	2
6	3.0	42:00	3
	0.5 (x4)	6:30 1:30 rest	2
7	4.0	56:00	3
	0.25 (x8)	3:30 1:00 rest	2
8	3.5	49:00	3
	2.0 (x3)	27:00	2

Week	Distance (miles)	Time Goal (minutes)	Frequency/Week (sessions)
9	4.0	54:00	3
	0.5 (x4)	6:30 1:30 rest	2
10	3.0	< 39:00	4–5

< means less than

Walking Exercise Programs (70+ years)
Beginner
Goal: 20:00/mile pace

Week	Distance (miles)	Time Goal (minutes)	Frequency/Week (sessions)
1	0.5	15:00	4–5
2	0.5	13:00	4–5
3	1.0	26:00	4–5
4	1.0	24:00	4–5
5	1.0	22:00	4–5
6	1.5	35:00	4–5
7	1.5	33:00	4–5
8	1.5	32:00	4–5
9	2.0	43:00	4–5
10	2.0	42:30	4–5
11	2.0	41:00	4–5
12	2.0	<40:00	4–5

< means less than

Recreational
Goal: 17:00/mile pace

Week	Distance (miles)	Time Goal (minutes)	Frequency/Week (sessions)
1	1.0	20:00	3–5
2	1.0	18:00	3–5
3	1.5	27:00	3–5
4	1.5	26:00	3–5
5	2.0	36:00	3–5
6	2.0	35:00	3–5
7	2.0	34:00	3–5
8	2.5	44:30	3–5
9	2.5	43:00	3–5
10	2.5	<42:30	3–5

< means less than

Elite (Race Walkers)
Goal: 15:00/mile pace

Week	Distance (miles)	Time Goal (minutes)	Frequency/Week (sessions)
1	1.5	30:00	5–6
2	1.5	27:00	5–6
3	2.0	36:00	5–6
4	2.0	34:00	5–6
5	2.5	42:30	5–6
6	2.5	40:00	5–6
7	3.0	49:00	5–6
8	3.0	47:00	5–6
9	3.0	46:00	5–6
10	3.0	<45:00	5–6

< means less than

GUIDE TO THE RUNNING/JOGGING PROGRAMS

1. To keep track of your distances, measure a flat, straight, curved, or rectangular surface equal to the mileage you expect to cover.

2. After a three- to five-minute warm-up of calisthenics or slow jogging, cover the prescribed distance at the beginning of the week, but don't worry too much about your speed. By the end of the week, attempt to reach the stated time goal. If you can't achieve the final goal, repeat the week.

3. Always cool down with slow walking for five minutes after completing the measured distance.

4. In the Beginner program, it's assumed that the exerciser has no previous aerobic conditioning.

5. The Recreational program has been structured for the exerciser who is already involved in a regular program and wants to improve his or her speed.

6. The Elite program is designed for the competitive exerciser. If a faster speed is desired and there are no medical restrictions, you can follow one of the programs for younger people. If you can't reach the top Elite levels, don't strain. Just exercise at a pace that is within your capacity.

7. By the final week of each program, an adequate level of aerobic conditioning will be reached. This level can be maintained on a schedule that involves four sessions per week. If you've reached the top level of the Beginner program and want to move on to the Recreational program, or if you've reached the top level in the Recreational program and want to try the Elite program, begin the next program at the lowest level indicated by the appropriate chart.

Running Where Jesus Walked

My longtime friend, collaborator, and patient, William Proctor, wrote these words a number of years ago after a trip to Israel:

When I set out on my run, the air was cool and crisp, and the sky was clear, with stars and moon still on the horizon. My first stop was the Garden of Gethsemane, just a couple of miles down the road. I really didn't expect to find the gates open, but I knew it would be only five minutes or so out of my way. So I decided to give it a try.

I ran straight down to the Damascus Gate, then along the wall of the old city past Herod's Gate, and then bore to the right, with the Mount of Olives on my left and the old city of Jerusalem on my right. The only person I encountered was an old Arab on a donkey who was urging his animal up a hill toward me. I went down a very steep incline into the Kidron Valley and crossed over in a few minutes to the Garden.

To my delight, the gates were open, and I walked in and stopped for a few minutes of prayer and meditation. The Garden of Gethsemane—all to myself! . . . As I prayed silently in this quiet garden, a sense of peace came over me.

—from William Proctor, "Running Where Jesus Walked,"
Christian Herald; April 1979, p. 30.

Lessons from Proctor's experience in Israel:

- Incorporate prayer and meditation into your endurance program.
- Use exercise during business or vacation trips as a means to explore new spiritual horizons.

---

8. An "x" in front of a number in parentheses in the Elite program refers to an interval training workout, a concept that involves covering relatively short distances in very fast times. Interval workouts are helpful in increasing race times. In week four of the up-to-forty-nine-years Elite program, for instance, the exerciser should first run three miles in twenty-three minutes. Then he should run three one-mile distances (indicated by "x3"), at a pace of 7:15 per mile, with a two-minute rest in between, as noted on the chart.

The one-half mile intervals are to be run in the specified times or at perceived exertion of "hard and heavy" effort. Quarter-mile intervals should be done in the specified times or at perceived exertion of "very hard," where you feel you can "still go on, but have to push."

9. All the programs can be used by men or women.

10. It's essential for every exerciser to secure medical clearance, including a stress electrocardiogram for men over forty and women over fifty, before beginning an exercise program. Beginning a program isn't recommended for anyone over age sixty *unless* adequate cardiovascular screening, including a stress ECG, has been accomplished and there are no signs or symptoms of heart disease. If you do begin at this age, you should have a thorough exam at least every two years.

Running/Jogging Exercise Programs (To 49 years)
Beginner
Goal: 8:00/mile pace

Week	Distance (miles)	Time Goal (minutes)	Frequency/Week (sessions)
1	2.0 (walk)	32:00	3–4
2	2.5 (walk)	40:00	3–4
3	3.0 (walk)	48:00	3–4
4	2.0 (walk/jog)	27:00	3–4
5	2.0 (walk/jog)	25:00	3–4
6	2.0 (jog)	24:00	3–4
7	2.0	22:00	4–5
8	2.0	20:00	4–5
9	3.0	26:00	4–5
10	3.0	25:00	4–5
11	3.0	24:00	4–5
12	3.0	<24:00	4

< means less than

Recreational
(conditioned runner wanting to increase speed)
Goal: 7:00/mile pace

Week	Distance (miles)	Time Goal (minutes)	Frequency/Week (sessions)
1	2.0	18:00	4–5
2	2.0	16:00	4–5
3	2.5	20:00	4–5
4	2.5	20:00	3
	0.5 (x3)	3:45 1:30 rest	2
5	3.0	24:00	2
	0.25 (x6)	1:30 1:00 rest	2
6	4.0	32:00	2
	0.5 (x4)	3:30 1:30 rest	3
7	3.0	22:00	3
	0.25 (x8)	1:30 1:00 rest	2
8	3.0	21:00	4–5

Elite
(competitive Masters runner)
Goal: 6:00 mile

Week	Distance (miles)	Time Goal (minutes)	Frequency/Week (sessions)
1	3.0	24:00	3
	2.0	15:30	2
2	3.0	23:45	2
	2.0	15:00	3
3	4.0	34:00	3
	0.5 (x3)	3:45 1:30 rest	2
4	3.0	23:00	3
	1.0 (x3)	7:15 2:00 rest	2
5	3.0	22:00	2
	0.5 (x4)	3:30	3
6	4.0	30:00	2
	0.25 (x8)	1:30 1:00 rest	2
7	3.0	21:00	3
	4.0	28:30	2
8	5.0	36:00	1
	2.0 (x3)	13:00 2:00 rest	2
		28:00	1
9	4.0	27:00	2
	0.5 (x4)	3:15	2
	5.0	35:00	1
10	3.0	18:30	1
	4.0	30:00	2
	1.0 (x2)	6:00 2:00 rest	1
11	3.0	18:15	2
	5.0	37:00	2
	0.25 (x8)	1:20 1:00 rest	1
12	3.0	<18:00	1
	4.0	28:00	2
	5.0	37:30	1

< means less than

Running/Jogging Exercise Programs (50–59 years)
Beginner
Goal: 10:00/mile pace

Week	Distance (miles)		Time Goal (minutes)	Frequency/Week (sessions)
1	1.0	(walk)	18:00	5
2	1.5	(walk)	27:00	4
3	2.0	(walk)	36:00	4
4	2.5	(walk)	45:00	4
5	3.0	(walk)	54:00	4
6	2.0	(walk/jog)	28:00	4
7	2.0	(walk/jog)	26:00	4
8	2.0	(jog)	24:00	4
9	2.5		30:00	4
10	2.5		28:00	4
11	2.5		27:00	4
12	3.0		33:00	4
13	3.0		31:30	4
14	3.0		< 30:00	4

< means less than

Recreational
(conditioned runner wanting to increase speed)
Goal: 9:00/mile pace

Week	Distance (miles)	Time Goal (minutes)	Frequency/Week (sessions)
1	2.0	20:00	4–5
2	2.0	19:00	4–5
3	2.0	18:00	4–5
4	2.5	23:45	4–5
5	2.5	23:15	4–5
6	2.5	22:30	4–5
7	3.0	28:30	4–5
8	3.0	28:00	4–5
9	3.0	27:30	4–5
10	3.0	< 27:00	4–5

< means less than

Elite
(competitive Masters runner)
Goal: 7:30 mile

Week	Distance (miles)	Time Goal (minutes)	Frequency/Week (sessions)
1	3.0	27:00	2
	2.0	18:00	3
2	3.0	26:00	4–5
3	4.0	36:00	2
	0.5 (x3)	4:15 1:30 rest	2
4	3.0	25:00	3
	1.0 (x3)	8:00 2:00 rest	2
5	4.0	34:00	3
	1.5 (x2)	12:00	2
6	3.0	24:00	3
	4.0	32:00	2
7	2.5 (x2)	20:00	2
	3.0	23:30	3
8	3.0	23:30	3
	0.5 (x4)	3:45 1:30 rest	2
9	3.0	23:00	3
	0.25 (x4)	1:40 1:00 rest	2
10	3.0	<22:30	4–5

< means less than

Running/Jogging Exercise Programs (60–69 years)
Beginner
Goal: 11:00/mile pace

Week	Distance (miles)	Time Goal (minutes)	Frequency/Week (sessions)
1	1.0 (walk)	20:00	5
2	1.0 (walk)	18:00	4
3	1.5 (walk)	28:00	4
4	1.5 (walk)	26:00	4
5	2.0 (walk)	36:00	4
6	2.0 (walk)	34:00	4
7	2.0 (walk/jog)	30:00	4
8	2.0 (walk/jog)	28:00	4
9	2.0 (walk/jog)	26:00	4
10	2.0 (jog)	24:00	4
11	2.0	23:00	4

Running/Jogging Exercise Programs (60–69 years)—Cont'd
Beginner
Goal: 11:00/mile pace

Week	Distance (miles)	Time Goal (minutes)	Frequency/Week (sessions)
12	2.0	22:00	4
13	2.5	28:00	4
14	2.5	27:15	4
15	2.5	<27:30	4

< means less than

Recreational
(conditioned runner wanting to increase speed)
Goal: 9:30/mile pace

Week	Distance (miles)	Time Goal (minutes)	Frequency/Week (sessions)
1	2.0	22:00	4–5
2	2.0	21:00	4–5
3	1.0 (x2)	9:45 2:00 rest	2
	2.0	20:00	3
4	2.5	26:00	4–5
5	2.5	25:00	4–5
6	2.5	24:30	4–5
7	3.0	30:00	4–5
8	1.5 (x2)	14:00 1:30 rest	2
	2.0	19:00	3
9	3.0	29:00	4
10	3.0	<28:30	4–5

< means less than

Elite
(competitive Masters runner)
Goal: 8:00/mile pace

Week	Distance (miles)	Time Goal (minutes)	Frequency/Week (sessions)
1	3.0	30:00	2
	2.0	19:45	3
2	4.0	40:00	4
3	3.5	35:00	4
4	2.0	19:00	2
	2.5	24:00	2

Week	Distance (miles)	Time Goal (minutes)	Frequency/Week (sessions)
5	3.0	28:30	4
6	4.0	36:00	2
	2.0	18:00	3
7	3.0	27:00	4
	1.0 (x2)	8:30 2:00 rest	1
8	2.0	17:00	2
	3.0	26:00	1
	1.0 (x2)	8:00 2:00 rest	2
9	2.0	16:30	1
	3.0	25:00	1
	0.5 (x3)	4:00	2
10	3.0	24:30	2
	2.0	16:00	1
11	1.0 (x3)	8:00 2:00 rest	2
	4.0	33:00	2
	3.0	24:00	2
12	3.0	<24:00	4–5

< means less than

Running/Jogging Exercise Programs (70+ years)
Beginner

Goal: 12:00/mile pace

Week	Distance (miles)	Time Goal (minutes)	Frequency/Week (sessions)
1	1.0 (walk)	24:00	5
2	1.0 (walk)	22:00	5
3	1.0 (walk)	20:00	5
4	1.5 (walk)	30:00	4
5	1.5 (walk)	28:00	4
6	1.5 (walk)	26:00	4
7	2.0 (walk)	38:00	4
8	2.0 (walk)	36:00	4
9	2.0 (walk/jog)	32:00	4
10	2.0 (walk/jog)	30:00	4
11	2.0 (walk/jog)	28:00	4
12	2.0 (jog)	27:00	4
13	2.0 (jog)	26:00	4
14	2.0 (jog)	25:00	4
15	2.0 (jog)	<24:00	4

< means less than

Recreational
(conditioned runner wanting to increase speed)
Goal: 10:00/mile

Week	Distance (miles)	Time Goal (minutes)	Frequency/Week (sessions)
1	2.0	25:00	4–5
2	2.0	24:00	4–5
3	1.0 (x2)	11:30 2:00 rest	2
	2.0	23:00	3
4	2.5	29:00	4–5
5	2.5	28:00	4–5
6	2.5	27:00	4–5
7	3.0	33:00	4–5
8	3.0	32:00	3
	1.5 (x2)	15:00	2
9	4.0	42:00	1
	2.5	26:00	4
10	2.0	20:00	2
	3.0	31:00	2
11	3.0	30:30	4–5
12	3.0	< 30:00	4–5

< means less than

Note: Elite program not recommended for this age group.

GUIDE TO THE TREADMILL PROGRAMS

1. After a three- to five-minute warm-up of calisthenics or of walking at two m.p.h., proceed with the workout, but don't worry too much about your speed. By the end of the week, attempt to reach the stated time goal. If you can't achieve the final goal, repeat the week. The program assumes that the treadmill is motor-driven, not self-propelled.

2. Always cool down with slow walking for five minutes at no incline after completing a workout.

3. In the Beginner program, it's assumed that the exerciser has no previous aerobic conditioning.

4. The Recreational program has been structured for the exerciser who is already involved in a regular program and wants to improve his or her speed.

5. The Elite program is designed for the competitive or highly experienced exerciser. If a faster speed is desired and there are no medical restrictions, you can follow one of the programs for younger people. If you can't

reach the top Elite levels, don't strain to try to do more. Just exercise at a pace that is within your capacity.

No specific treadmill program has been provided for the Elite, competitive race walker or runner past seventy years of age. Training in this age group must be closely supervised on an individual basis. After clearance by a thorough medical exam, with stress test, the experienced over-seventy athlete can proceed with a treadmill program at one of the younger age levels.

6. By the final week of each program, an adequate level of endurance conditioning will be reached. This level can be maintained on a schedule that involves four sessions per week. If you've reached the top level of the Beginner program and want to move on to the Recreational program, or if you've reached the top level in the Recreational program and want to try the Elite program, begin the next program at the lowest level indicated by the chart.

7. All the programs can be used by men or women.

8. It's essential for every exerciser to secure medical clearance, including a stress electrocardiogram, before beginning an exercise program. Beginning a program isn't recommended for anyone over age sixty unless adequate cardiovascular screening, including a stress ECG, has been accomplished and there are no signs or symptoms of heart disease. If you do begin at this age, you should have a thorough exam every two years.

Treadmill Exercise Programs (To 49 years)
Beginner
(walking only)
Max speed: 14:00/mile

Week	Speed (mph)	Incline (%)	Time Goal (minutes)	Frequency/Week (sessions)
1	3.0	0	20:00	4–5
2	3.0	0	25:00	4–5
3	3.25	0	30:00	4–5
4	3.25	2.5	30:00	4–5
5	3.5	2.5	25:00	4–5
6	3.5	2.5	30:00	4–5
7	3.75	2.5	25:00	4–5
8	3.75	5	30:00	4–5
9	4.0	5	25:00	4–5
10	4.0	5	30:00	4–5
11	4.25	7.5	25:00	4–5
12	4.25	7.5	30:00	4–5

Recreational
(aerobic walking and slow jogging)
Max speed: 12:00/mile

Week	Speed (mph)	Incline (%)	Time Goal (minutes)	Frequency/Week (sessions)
1	4.0	0	20:00	4–5
2	4.0	0	30:00	4–5
3	4.0	2	30:00	4–5
4	4.0	5	30:00	4–5
5	4.5	0	30:00	4–5
6	4.5	2.5	30:00	4–5
7	4.5	5	30:00	4–5
8	5.0	0	24:00	4–5
9	5.0	2.5	24:00	4–5
10	5.0	5	24:00	4–5

Elite
(race walker or experienced runner)
Max speed: 8:00/mile

Week	Speed (mph)	Incline (%)	Time Goal (minutes)	Frequency/Week (sessions)
1	4.0	0	30:00	4–5
2	4.5	0	30:00	4–5
3	5.0	0	25:00	4–5
4	5.5	0	25:00	4–5
5	6.0*	0	25:00	4–5
6	6.0	0	30:00	4–5
7	6.5	0	20:00	4–5
8**	6.5	0	25:00	4–5
9	7.0	0	20:00	4–5
10	7.0	0	25:00	4–5
11	7.5	0	25:00	4–5
12	7.5	0	24:00	4–5

*Probable maximum speed for race walking.

**Beginning with week 8, the following inclines can be used to increase the workload and the aerobic benefits of running.

Week	Incline (%)
8	2.5
9	2.5
10	5
11	5
12	7.5

Treadmill Exercise Programs (50–59 years)
Beginner
(walking only)
Max speed: 15:00/mile

Week	Speed (mph)	Incline (%)	Time Goal (minutes)	Frequency/Week (sessions)
1	3.0	0	20:00	4–5
2	3.0	0	25:00	4–5
3	3.0	0	30:00	4–5
4	3.25	0	30:00	4–5
5	3.25	2.5	30:00	4–5
6	3.50	5	30:00	4–5
7	3.50	2.5	30:00	4–5
8	3.50	5	30:00	4–5
9	3.75	2.5	30:00	4–5
10	3.75	5	30:00	4–5
11	4.0	2.5	30:00	4–5
12	4.0	5	30:00	4–5

Recreational
(aerobic walking and slow jogging)
Max speed: 13:20/mile

Week	Speed (mph)	Incline (%)	Time Goal (minutes)	Frequency/Week (sessions)
1	3.5	0	20:00	4–5
2	4.0	0	20:00	4–5
3	4.0	0	25:00	4–5
4	4.0	2.5	30:00	4–5
5	4.25	0	30:00	4–5
6	4.25	2.5	30:00	4–5

Recreational—Cont'd
(aerobic walking and slow jogging)
Max speed: 13:20/mile

Week	Speed (mph)	Incline (%)	Time Goal (minutes)	Frequency/Week (sessions)
7	4.25	5	30:00	4–5
8	4.5	0	28:00	4–5
9	4.5	2.5	28:00	4–5
10	4.5	5	27:00	4–5

Elite
(race walker or experienced runner)
Max speed: 8:30/mile

Week	Speed (mph)	Incline (%)	Time Goal (minutes)	Frequency/Week (sessions)
1	3.5	0	25:00	4–5
2	4.0	0	30:00	4–5
3	4.0	0	30:00	4–5
4	5.0	0	25:00	4–5
5	5.0	0	25:00	4–5
6	5.5	0	25:00	4–5
7	5.5	0	30:00	4–5
8**	6.0*	0	30:00	4–5
9	6.0	0	30:00	4–5
10	6.5	0	25:00	4–5
11	6.5	0	25:00	4–5
12	7.0	0	25:30	4–5

*Probable maximum speed for race walking.
**Beginning with week 8, the following inclines can be used to increase the workload and the aerobic benefits of running.

Week	Incline (%)
8	2.5
9	2.5
10	2.5
11	5
12	5

Treadmill Exercise Programs (60–69 years)
Beginner
(walking only)
Max speed: 16:00/mile

Week	Speed (mph)	Incline (%)	Time Goal (minutes)	Frequency/Week (sessions)
1	2.5	0	20:00	3–4
2	2.5	0	25:00	3–4
3	3.0	0	25:00	3–4
4	3.0	0	25:00	3–4
5	3.0	0	25:00	3–4
6	3.25	0	25:00	3–4
7	3.25	2.5	25:00	3–4
8	3.25	2.5	30:00	3–4
9	3.50	2.5	25:00	3–4
10	3.50	5	30:00	3–4
11	3.75	2.5	30:00	3–4
12	3.75	5	32:00	4

Recreational
(aerobic walking and slow jogging)
Max speed: 14:00/mile

Week	Speed (mph)	Incline (%)	Time Goal (minutes)	Frequency/Week (sessions)
1	3.0	0	15:00	4–5
2	3.5	0	20:00	4–5
3	3.5	0	25:00	4–5
4	3.75	2.5	25:00	4–5
5	3.75	5	30:00	4–5
6	4.0	2.5	25:00	4–5
7	4.0	5	30:00	4–5
8	4.25	0	25:00	4–5
9	4.25	2.5	25:00	4–5
10	4.25	5	28:00	4–5

Elite
(race walker or experienced runner)
Max speed: 9:00/mile

Week	Speed (mph)	Incline (%)	Time Goal (minutes)	Frequency/Week (sessions)
1	3.0	0	25:00	4–5
2	3.5	0	30:00	4–5
3	4.0	0	30:00	4–5
4	4.5	0	25:00	4–5
5	4.5	0	30:00	4–5
6	5.0	0	30:00	4–5
7	5.5	0	30:00	4–5
8**	6.0*	0	30:00	4–5
9	6.0	0	32:00	4–5
10	6.5	0	28:00	4–5
11	6.5	0	30:00	4–5
12	6.75	0	27:00	4–5

*Probable maximum speed for race walking.

**Beginning with week 8, the following inclines can be used to increase the workload and the aerobic benefits of running.

Week	Incline (%)
8	2
9	2.5
10	2.5
11	5
12	5

Treadmill Exercise Programs (70+ years)
Beginner
(walking only)
Max speed: 20:00/mile

Week	Speed (mph)	Incline (%)	Time Goal (minutes)	Frequency/Week (sessions)
1	2.0	0	15:00	3–4
2	2.0	0	20:00	3–4
3	2.25	0	20:00	3–4

Week	Speed (mph)	Incline (%)	Time Goal (minutes)	Frequency/Week (sessions)
4	2.25	0	25:00	3–4
5	2.50	0	20:00	3–4
6	2.50	2.5	25:00	3–4
7	2.50	5	25:00	3–4
8	2.75	0	20:00	3–4
9	2.75	2.5	25:00	3–4
10	2.75	5	30:00	3–4
11	3.0	2.5	25:00	3–4
12	3.0	5	30:00	4

Recreational
(aerobic walking and slow jogging)
Max speed: 15:00/mile

Week	Speed (mph)	Incline (%)	Time Goal (minutes)	Frequency/Week (sessions)
1	2.5	0	15:00	4–5
2	2.5	0	20:00	4–5
3	3.0	0	20:00	4–5
4	3.0	0	25:00	4–5
5	3.5	2.5	20:00	4–5
6	3.5	5	25:00	4–5
7	3.75	2.5	20:00	4–5
8	3.75	5	25:00	4–5
9	4.0	2.5	25:00	4–5
10	4.0	5	30:00	4–5

Note: Elite program not recommended for this age group.

GUIDELINES TO THE OUTDOOR CYCLING PROGRAMS

1. Go through the usual three- to five-minute warm-up of calisthenics or slow cycling. As you move into the main part of the workout, speeds and times will vary, depending on wind velocity, road surface, and weather conditions. Drafting (riding close behind) other cyclists will help you develop speed.

2. Recreational and Elite programs assume that the individual has already established a cycling base of forty miles per week or more. Some weeks are designed to be easier workouts to give your legs a "recovery week" about every four weeks.

3. Interval workouts of three-mile lengths should be preceded by a ten- to fifteen-minute cycling warm-up. The three-minute rest or recovery

should include easy spinning at less than 100 r.p.m. (revolutions per minute) to allow yourself enough time to recoup and keep your intervals at consistent times. A single revolution consists of one 360-degree turn of one of your pedals. Also, the interval workouts are indicated by a "times" sign, an "x," followed by the number of workouts per session.

4. Cool down and stretch upon completion of all cycling workouts.

5. In normal aerobic cycling, try to maintain r.p.m. of eighty-five to ninety. When climbing hills, try to maintain more than seventy-five r.p.m. by using lower gears.

6. All programs assume that the cyclist will be using a bicycle with three or more gears. For a cyclist over sixty and especially over seventy, a large-wheeled bike or even three-wheeled adult tricycle is recommended for safety.

7. By the final week of each program, an adequate level of endurance conditioning will be reached. This level can be maintained on a schedule that involves three to four sessions per week.

8. The program can be used by men or women.

9. It's essential for every exerciser to secure medical clearance, including a stress electrocardiogram, before beginning an exercise program. Beginning an interval program isn't recommended for anyone over sixty years of age *unless* adequate cardiovascular screening, including a stress ECG, has been accomplished and there are no signs or symptoms of heart disease. If you do begin at this age, you should have a thorough exam every two years.

Outdoor Cycling Programs (To 49 years)
Beginner
Goal: 15 mph pace for 15 miles or farther

Week	Speed (mph)	Distance (miles)	Time Goal (minutes)	Frequency/Week (sessions)
1	12.4	6	29:00	3–4
2	13.0	8	37:00	3–4
3	13.7	8	35:00	3–4
4	14.0	8	34:20	2
	13.8	12	52:00	2
5	14.25	10	42:15	4
6	14.6	10	41:00	3
	14.0	15	64:20	1
7	15.0	10	40:00	1
	14.3	15	63:00	1
	14.1	18	76:30	1

Week	Speed (mph)	Distance (miles)	Time Goal (minutes)	Frequency/Week (sessions)
8	15.2	10	39:30	1
	14.5	15	62:00	1
	14.0	20	85:45	1
9	15.4	10	39:00	1
	15.25	15	61:00	1
	14.4	20	83:30	1
10	15.75	10	38:00	1
	15.0	15	60:00	1
	14.0	24	103:00	1
11	16.0	10	37:30	2
	15.25	15	59:00	2
12	16.0	10	37:30	1
	15.25	15	59:00	1
	14.5	25	103:30	1

Recreational

Goal: 18 mph pace for 20 miles or farther

Week	Speed (mph)	Distance (miles)	Time Goal (minutes)	Frequency/Week (sessions)
1	15.0	10	40:00	2
	15.0	15	60:00	1
2	15.0	12	48:00	2
	15.0	18	72:00	1
3	15.5	15	58:00	2
	15.4	20	78:00	1
4	16.0	12	45:00	3
	15.8	20	76:00	1
5	16.5	15	54:30	2
	16.0	27	101:00	1
6	17.0	15	53:00	3
	16.5	20	73:00	1
7	18.6	3 (x3)	9:40 3:00 rest	1
	17.5	15	51:30	2
	16.8	20	71:30	1
8	18.9	3 (x3)	9:30 3:00 rest	1
	17.8	18	60:40	1
	16.5	30	109:00	1

Recreational—Cont'd
Goal: 18 mph pace for 20 miles or farther

Week	Speed (mph)	Distance (miles)	Time Goal (minutes)		Frequency/Week (sessions)
9	19.0	3 (x4)	9:28	3:00 rest	1
	18.0	15	50:00		2
	17.1	20	70:00		1
10	19.3	3 (x4)	9:20	3:00 rest	1
	18.4	15	49:00		2
	18.0	20	66:40		1

Elite
(Master cyclist)
Goal: 21–23 mph pace for 20 miles or farther

Week	Speed (mph)	Distance (miles)	Time Goal (minutes)		Frequency/Week (sessions)
1	17.5	15	51:25		2
	17.0	25	87:00		1
2	20.0	3 (x4)	9:00	3:00 rest	1
	18.0	15	50:00		2
	18.5	20	65:00		1
3	20.4	3 (x4)	8:50	3:00 rest	1
	18.5	25	81:00		1
	19.2	20	62:30		2
4	20.8	3 (x5)	8:40	3:00 rest	1
	19.2	30	94:00		1
	19.7	20	61:00		2
5	21.2	3 (x5)	8:30	3:00 rest	1
	18.8	22	70:00		1
	20.0	20	60:00		1
6	21.6	3 (x5)	8:20	3:00 rest	1
	19.6	30	92:00		1
	20.2	20	59:30		2
7	21.8	3 (x5)	8:15	3:00 rest	1
	20.0	30	90:00		1
	20.4	20	58:45		2
8	22.2	3 (x5)	8:05	3:00 rest	1
	20.2	30	89:00		1
	20.7	20	58:00		2
9	20.0	15	45:00		2
	19.5	40	123:00		1

Week	Speed (mph)	Distance (miles)	Time Goal (minutes)	Frequency/Week (sessions)
10	22.5	3 (x6)	8:00 3:00 rest	1
	20.7	30	87:00	1
	21.0	20	57:00	2
11	22.7	3 (x5)	7:55 3:00 rest	1
	20.3	40	118:00	1
	21.4	20	56:00	2
12	23.0	3 (x6)	7:50 3:00 rest	1
	21.0	30	85:30	1
	20.7	25	72:30	1
	22.0	20	54:30	1

Outdoor Cycling Programs (50–59 years)
Beginner

Goal: 14 mph pace for 15 miles or farther

Week	Speed (mph)	Distance (miles)	Time Goal (minutes)	Frequency/Week (sessions)
1	10.0	5	30:00	3–4
2	11.0	6	32:45	3–4
3	11.5	7	36:35	3–4
4	11.5	8	41:45	3–4
5	12.0	8	40:00	2
	11.5	10	52:15	2
6	12.0	10	50:00	4
7	12.5	8	38:25	3
	11.5	12	62:40	1
8	13.0	8	37:00	1
	12.5	10	48:00	1
	12.0	15	75:00	1
9	14.0	10	43:00	1
	13.0	15	69:15	1
	13.0	16	73:55	1
10	15.0	8	32:00	1
	13.5	15	66:20	1
	14.0	10	42:55	1
11	15.0	10	40:00	1
	14.5	12	49:40	1
	13.5	17	75:30	1
12	14.0	15	64:20	2
	13.5	17.5	77:45	1

Recreational

Goal: 17.5 mph pace for 15 miles or farther

Week	Speed (mph)	Distance (miles)	Time Goal (minutes)	Frequency/Week (sessions)
1	12.5	8	38:24	3–4
2	12.5	9	43:12	3–4
3	12.5	10	48:00	2
	12.5	12	57:42	2
4	15.0	8	32:00	3
	12.0	14	70:00	1
5	15.0	12	48:00	2
	12.5	13	62:24	2
6	16.0	10	37:30	3
	12.5	15	72:00	1
7	18.0	3 (x3)	10:00 3:00 rest	1
	15.0	10	40:00	1
	14.0	12	51:30	2
8	16.5	14	51:00	2
	13.0	16	74:00	2
9	20.0	3 (x3)	9:00 3:00 rest	1
	17.5	8	27:30	2
	16.5	16	58:15	1
10	18.0	12	40:00	2
	17.5	15	51:30	2

Elite

(Master cyclist)

Goal: 20 mph pace for 20 miles or farther

Week	Speed (mph)	Distance (miles)	Time Goal (minutes)	Frequency/Week (sessions)
1	16.0	10	37:30	2
	15.0	15	60:00	2
2	18.0	3 (x3)	10:00 3:00 rest	1
	16.0	12.5	46:50	2
	16.0	15	56:15	1
3	16.5	15	54:24	2
	17.0	12	42:20	2

Week	Speed (mph)	Distance (miles)	Time Goal (minutes)	Frequency/Week (sessions)
4	19.0	3 (x4)	9:30	1
	17.0	15	53:00	2
	17.0	17.5	61:45	1
5	20.0	3 (x4)	9:00 3:00 rest	1
	18.0	10	33:20	2
	17.0	20	70:45	1
6	21.0	3 (x5)	8:48 3:00 rest	1
	19.0	12.5	39:30	2
	18.5	15	48:35	1
7	20.0	15	45:00	2
	18.0	20	66:35	2
8	22.0	3 (x5)	8:12	1
	20.0	15	45:00	2
	18.0	22	73:20	1
9	20.0	17.5	52:30	2
	19.0	20	63:15	2
10	22.0	3 (x6)	8:12	1
	19.0	20	63:15	2
	18.0	25	83:15	1
11	22.0	3 (x6)	8:12	1
	18.5	25	81:00	2
12	20.0	20	60:00	2
	18.5	25	81:00	2

Outdoor Cycling Programs (60–69 years)
Beginner
Goal: 12 mph pace for 12 miles or farther

Week	Speed (mph)	Distance (miles)	Time Goal (minutes)	Frequency/Week (sessions)
1	8.0	4	30:00	3–4
2	9.0	5	33:20	3–4
3	10.0	6	36:00	3–4
4	10.5	7	40:00	3–4
5	11.0	8	43:45	3–4
6	11.5	8	41:50	2
	10.5	10	57:00	2

Outdoor Cycling Programs (60–69 years)—Cont'd
Beginner
Goal: 12 mph pace for 12 miles or farther

Week	Speed (mph)	Distance (miles)	Time Goal (minutes)	Frequency/Week (sessions)
7	12.0	8	40:00	3
	11.0	12	65:25	1
8	12.5	7	33:45	1
	12.0	9	45:00	1
	11.5	10	52:15	1
9	12.5	8	38:25	1
	12.0	10	50:00	1
	11.5	12	62:40	1
10	12.5	10	48:00	1
	11.5	12	62:40	1
	13.0	8	37:00	1
11	11.5	12	62:40	2
	13.0	10	46:10	1
12	12.0	12	60:00	2
	11.0	15	81:45	1

Recreational
Goal: 14.5 mph pace for 15 miles or farther

Week	Speed (mph)	Distance (miles)	Time Goal (minutes)	Frequency/Week (sessions)
1	10.0	6	36:00	3–4
2	10.0	8	48:00	3–4
3	10.0	9	54:00	3–4
4	10.0	10	60:00	2
	12.5	8	38:25	2
5	12.5	10	48:00	2
	14.0	10	43:00	2
6	16.0	3 (x3)	11:15	1
	14.0	12	51:30	1
	15.0	10	40:00	2
7	14.5	12	49:40	2
	13.5	14	62:10	2
8	17.5	3 (x3)	10:20 3:00 rest	1
	14.0	15	64:20	1
	15.0	10	40:00	2

Week	Speed (mph)	Distance (miles)	Time Goal (minutes)	Frequency/Week (sessions)
9	15.0	12	48:00	2
	14.0	16	68:40	2
10	15.0	12	48:00	2
	14.5	15	62:10	2

Elite
(Master cyclist)
Goal: 16 mph pace for 15 miles or farther

Week	Speed (mph)	Distance (miles)	Time Goal (minutes)	Frequency/Week (sessions)
1	12.0	8	40:00	2
	12.0	10	50:00	2
2	13.0	10	46:15	2
	12.0	12.5	63:30	2
3	16.0	3 (x3)	11:15	1
	13.5	10	44:25	2
	14.0	12.5	53:40	2
4	13.0	15	69:20	2
	14.0	10	42:55	2
5	18.0	2 (x4)	6:40	1
	14.0	10	42:55	2
	14.5	12	49:40	1
6	18.0	2 (x5)	6:40	1
	15.0	12.5	50:00	2
	14.0	15.0	64:20	1
7	15.0	12.5	50:00	2
	14.5	15	62:10	2
8	20.0	2 (x6)	6:00	1
	14.5	10	41:25	2
	14.0	16	68:40	1
9	15.0	15	60:00	2
	14.0	17	72:55	2
10	18.0	3 (x4)	10:00	1
	16.5	12	43:40	2
	14.0	18	77:15	1
11	19.0	3 (x4)	9:30	1
	15.5	15	59:30	2
	15.0	16	64:00	1
12	16.0	15	56:15	2
	12.5	20	96:00	1

Outdoor Cycling Programs (70+ years)
Beginner
Goal: 10 mph pace for 10 miles or farther

Week	Speed (mph)	Distance (miles)	Time Goal (minutes)	Frequency/Week (sessions)
1	7.5	4	32:00	3–4
2	8.0	4	30:00	3–4
3	8.5	5	35:20	3–4
4	9.0	5	33:20	3–4
5	9.5	6	38:00	3–4
6	9.5	7	44:15	3–4
7	10.0	7	42:00	2
	9.5	8	50:40	2
8	10.5	8	45:45	3
	9.0	10	66:42	1
9	9.5	10	63:15	3
10	9.5	8	50:40	1
	9.5	9	56:50	1
	9.5	10	63:10	1
11	9.0	12	80:00	2
	10.0	8	48:00	1
12	10.0	10	60:00	2
	9.5	12	75:55	1

Recreational
Goal: 12.5 mph pace for 12 miles or farther

Week	Speed (mph)	Distance (miles)	Time Goal (minutes)	Frequency/Week (sessions)
1	8.0	5	37:30	3–4
2	9.0	6	40:00	3–4
3	10.0	7	42:00	3–4
4	10.0	8	48:00	2
	10.0	10	60:00	2
5	10.5	10	57:00	2
	10.5	10	57:00	2
6	14.0	3 (x3)	12:45 3:00 rest	1
	10.0	12	72:00	2
	12.0	8	40:00	1

Week	Speed (mph)	Distance (miles)	Time Goal (minutes)	Frequency/Week (sessions)
7	12.0	10	50:00	2
	11.0	12	65:25	2
8	15.0	2 (x4)	8:00 3:00 rest	1
	14.0	8	34:20	2
	11.0	14	76:20	1
9	12.5	10	48:00	2
	12.0	12	60:00	2
10	12.5	12	57:45	3
	10.0	15	90:00	1

Note: Elite program not recommended for this age group.

GUIDE TO THE STATIONARY CYCLING PROGRAMS

1. Warm up before beginning the actual workout by doing light calisthenics or cycling for about five minutes at seventeen to twenty m.p.h. (sixty-five to seventy-five r.p.m., or revolutions per minute), without resistance on the bike. At the conclusion of the exercise, cool down by cycling for five minutes with no resistance.

2. Adjust the resistance on the bike so that when you are pedaling, your Rate of Perceived Exertion (RPE), as described on page 79, is at a level that you consider "somewhat hard" to "hard."

A more precise option, which is preferred by many experienced stationary cyclists, is to add enough resistance to the bike so that your pulse rate (PR), counted for ten seconds immediately after exercise and multiplied by six, equals the specified rate in the charts. If your pulse is higher than the specified rate, lower the resistance before you cycle again. If your pulse rate is lower, add resistance to the bike.

3. In the Beginner program, it's assumed that the exerciser has no previous aerobic conditioning.

4. The Recreational program has been structured for the exerciser who is already involved in a regular program and wants to improve his or her speed.

5. The Elite program is designed for the competitive or highly experienced exerciser. If a faster speed is desired and there are no medical restrictions, you can follow one of the programs for younger people. If you can't reach the top Elite levels, don't strain. Just exercise at a pace that is within your capacity.

No specific program has been provided for the Elite, competitive cycler past seventy years of age. Training in this age group must be closely supervised on an individual basis. After clearance by a thorough medical exam, with stress test, the experienced over-seventy athlete can proceed with an appropriate program at one of the younger age levels.

6. By the final week of each program, an adequate level of aerobic conditioning will be reached. This level can be maintained on a schedule that involves four sessions per week. If you've reached the top level of the Beginner program and want to move on to the Recreational program, or if you've reached the top level in the Recreational program and want to try the Elite program, begin the next program at the lowest level indicated by the chart.

7. All the programs can be used by men or women.

8. It's essential for exercisers to secure medical clearance, including a stress electrocardiogram, before beginning an exercise program. Beginning a program isn't recommended for anyone over age sixty *unless* adequate cardiovascular screening, including a stress ECG, has been accomplished and there are no signs or symptoms of heart disease. If you do begin at this age, you should have a thorough exam every two years.

Stationary Cycling Exercise Programs (To 49 years)

Beginner

Week	Speed (mph/rpm)	Time Goal (minutes)	Pulse Rate (after exercise)	Frequency/Week (sessions)
1	15.0/55	6:00	<140	4–5
2	15.0/55	8:00	<140	4–5
3	15.0/55	10:00	<140	4–5
4	15.0/55	12:00	<150	4–5
5	15.0/55	14:00	<150	4–5
6	15.0/55	16:00	<150	4–5
7	15.0/55	18:00	<150	4–5
8	15.0/55	20:00	<150	4–5
9	17.5/65	20:00	<150	4–5
10	17.5/65	22:00	>150	4–5
11	20.0/75	22:00	>150	4–5
12	20.0/75	25:00	>150	4–5
13	20.0/75	27:30	>150	4–5
14	25.0/90+	30:00	>150	4–5

< means less than
> means more than

Recreational
(already involved in a program but wanting to improve fitness)

Week	Speed (mph/rpm)	Time Goal (minutes)	Pulse Rate (after exercise)	Frequency/Week (sessions)
1	22.0/80	20:00	>150	4–5
2	22.0/80	25:00	>150	4–5
3	22.0/80	30:00	>150	4–5
4	25.0/90	20:00	>150	4–5
5	25.0/90	25:00	>150	4–5
6	25.0/90	30:00	>150	4–5
7	26.5/95	25:00	>160	4–5
8	26.5/95	30:00	>160	4–5
9	26.5/95	35:00	>160	4–5
10	26.5/95+	40:00	>160	4–5

> means more than

Elite
(competitive Masters cyclist interested in fitness and/or speed)

Week	Speed (mph/rpm)	Time Goal (minutes)	Pulse Rate (after exercise)	Frequency/Week (sessions)
1	25.0/ 90	30:00	>150	4–5
2	25.0/ 90	35:00	>150	4–5
3	25.0/ 90	40:00	>150	4–5
4	25.0/ 90	45:00	>150	4–5
5	28.5/100	35:00	>160	4–5
6	28.5/100	40:00	>160	4–5
7	28.5/100	45:00	>160	4–5
8	32.5/110	35:00	>160	4–5
9	32.5/110	40:00	>160	4–5
10	32.5/110	45:00	>160	4–5

> means more than

Stationary Cycling Exercise Programs (50–59 years)
Beginner

Week	Speed (mph/rpm)	Time Goal (minutes)	Pulse Rate (after exercise)	Frequency/Week (sessions)
1	15.0/55	6:00	<135	4–5
2	15.0/55	8:00	<135	4–5
3	15.0/55	10:00	<135	4–5
4	15.0/55	12:00	<140	4–5

Stationary Cycling Exercise Programs (50–59 years)—Cont'd
Beginner

Week	Speed (mph/rpm)	Time Goal (minutes)	Pulse Rate (after exercise)	Frequency/Week (sessions)
5	15.0/55	14:00	<140	4–5
6	17.5/65	16:00	<140	4–5
7	17.5/65	18:00	<140	4–5
8	17.5/65	20:00	<140	4–5
9	20.0/75	20:00	<150	4–5
10	20.0/75	20:00	<150	4–5
11	20.0/75	22:00	<150	4–5
12	25.0/90	22:00	<150	4–5
13	25.0/90	25:00	>150	4–5
14	25.0/90	30:00	>150	4–5

< means less than
> means more than

Recreational
(already involved in a program but wanting to improve)

Week	Speed (mph/rpm)	Time Goal (minutes)	Pulse Rate (after exercise)	Frequency/Week (sessions)
1	20.0/75	20:00	>140	4–5
2	20.0/75	25:00	>140	4–5
3	20.0/75	30:00	>140	4–5
4	21.5/80	20:00	>140	4–5
5	21.5/80	25:00	>140	4–5
6	21.5/80	30:00	>140	4–5
7	23.0/85	25:00	>150	4–5
8	23.0/85	30:00	>150	4–5
9	23.0/85	35:00	>150	4–5
10	25.0/90+	40:00	>150	4–5

> means more than

Elite
(competitive Masters cyclist interested in fitness and/or speed)

Week	Speed (mph/rpm)	Time Goal (minutes)	Pulse Rate (after exercise)	Frequency/Week (sessions)
1	22.5/ 80	30:00	>140	4–5
2	21.5/ 80	35:00	>140	4–5
3	21.5/ 80	40:00	>140	4–5

Week	Speed (mph/rpm)	Time Goal (minutes)	Pulse Rate (after exercise)	Frequency/Week (sessions)
4	21.5/ 80	45:00	>140	4–5
5	25.0/ 90	35:00	>150	4–5
6	25.0/ 90	40:00	>150	4–5
7	25.0/ 90	45:00	>150	4–5
8	28.5/100	35:00	>150	4–5
9	28.5/100	40:00	>150	4–5
10	28.5/100	45:00	>160	4–5

> means more than

Stationary Cycling Exercise Programs (60–69 years)

Beginner

Week	Speed (mph/rpm)	Time Goal (minutes)	Pulse Rate (after exercise)	Frequency/Week (sessions)
1	15.0/55	4:00	>120	4–5
2	15.0/55	6:00	>120	4–5
3	15.0/55	8:00	>120	4–5
4	15.0/55	10:00	>120	4–5
5	15.0/55	12:00	>130	4–5
6	15.0/55	14:00	>130	4–5
7	15.0/55	16:00	>130	4–5
8	17.5/65	18:00	>130	4–5
9	17.5/65	20:00	>130	4–5
10	17.5/65	22:30	>140	4–5
11	20.0/75	25:00	>140	4–5
12	20.0/75	26:00	>140	4–5
13	20.0/75	28:00	>140	4–5
14	20.0/75	30:00	>140	4–5

> means more than

Recreational

(already involved in a program but wanting to improve fitness)

Week	Speed (mph/rpm)	Time Goal (minutes)	Pulse Rate (after exercise)	Frequency/Week (sessions)
1	20.0/75	15:00	>130	4–5
2	20.0/75	20:00	>130	4–5
3	20.0/75	25:00	>130	4–5
4	20.0/75	30:00	>130	4–5

Recreational—Cont'd

(already involved in a program but wanting to improve fitness)

Week	Speed (mph/rpm)	Time Goal (minutes)	Pulse Rate (after exercise)	Frequency/Week (sessions)
5	21.5/80	25:00	>140	4–5
6	21.5/80	25:00	>140	4–5
7	21.5/80	30:00	>140	4–5
8	23.0/85	30:00	>140	4–5
9	23.0/85	30:00	>140	4–5
10	23.0/85	35:00	>140	4–5

> means more than

Elite

(competitive Masters cyclist wanting fitness and/or speed)

Week	Speed (mph/rpm)	Time Goal (minutes)	Pulse Rate (after exercise)	Frequency/Week (sessions)
1	20.0/75	30:00	>130	4–5
2	20.0/75	35:00	>130	4–5
3	20.0/75	40:00	>130	4–5
4	20.0/75	45:00	>130	4–5
5	21.5/80	35:00	>140	4–5
6	21.5/80	40:00	>140	4–5
7	21.5/80	45:00	>140	4–5
8	25.0/90	35:00	>140	4–5
9	25.0/90	40:00	>140	4–5
10	25.0/90	45:00	>150	4–5

> means more than

Stationary Cycling Exercise Programs (70+ years)

Beginner

Week	Speed (mph/rpm)	Time Goal (minutes)	Pulse Rate (after exercise)	Frequency/Week (sessions)
1	15.0/55	4:00	>100	4–5
2	15.0/55	6:00	>100	4–5
3	15.0/55	8:00	>100	4–5
4	15.0/55	10:00	>100	4–5
5	15.0/55	12:00	>110	4–5
6	15.0/55	14:00	>110	4–5
7	15.0/55	16:00	>110	4–5

Week	Speed (mph/rpm)	Time Goal (minutes)	Pulse Rate (after exercise)	Frequency/Week (sessions)
8	16.5/60	18:00	>110	4–5
9	16.5/60	20:00	>110	4–5
10	16.5/60	22:00	>120	4–5
11	17.5/65	24:00	>120	4–5
12	17.5/65	26:00	>120	4–5
13	17.5/65	28:00	>120	4–5
14	17.5/65	30:00	>120	4–5

> means more than

Recreational

(already involved in a program but wanting to improve fitness)

Week	Speed (mph/rpm)	Time Goal (minutes)	Pulse Rate (after exercise)	Frequency/Week (sessions)
1	16.5/60	15:00	>120	4–5
2	16.5/60	20:00	>120	4–5
3	16.5/60	25:00	>120	4–5
4	16.5/60	30:00	>120	4–5
5	20.0/75	25:00	>130	4–5
6	20.0/75	25:00	>130	4–5
7	20.0/75	30:00	>130	4–5
8	21.5/80	30:00	>130	4–5
9	21.5/80	30:00	>130	4–5
10	23.5/85	30:00	>130	4–5

> means more than

Note: Elite program not recommended for this age group.

GUIDE TO THE SWIMMING PROGRAMS

1. Use any stroke that enables you to swim the required distance in the alloted time. Resting is permitted during the initial weeks. The objective is to reach the distance-time goals at the end of a week.

2. After a three- to five-minute warm-up of calisthenics or slow swimming, cover the prescribed distance at the beginning of the week, but don't worry too much about your speed. By the end of the week, attempt to reach the stated time goal. If you can't achieve the final goal, repeat the week.

3. Always cool down with slow swimming for five minutes after completing the measured distance.

4. In the Beginner program, it's assumed that the exerciser has no previous aerobic conditioning.

5. The Recreational program has been structured for the exerciser who is already involved in a regular program and wants to improve his or her speed.

6. The Elite program is designed for the competitive exerciser. If a faster speed is desired and there are no medical restrictions, you can follow one of the programs for younger people. If you can't reach the top Elite levels, don't strain. Just exercise at a pace that is within your capacity.

7. By the final week of each program, an adequate level of endurance conditioning will be reached. This level can be maintained on a schedule that involves three to four sessions per week. If you've reached the top level of the Beginner program and want to move on to the Recreational program, or if you've reached the top level in the Recreational program and want to try the Elite program, begin the next program at the lowest level indicated by the chart.

9. An "x" in front of a number in parentheses in the Elite program refers to an interval training workout, a concept that involves covering relatively short distance in very fast times. Interval workouts are helpful in increasing race times.

10. All the programs can be used by men or women, but for women to maintain their bone mineral content (and prevent osteoporosis), it's necessary to swim at least three hours per week.

11. It's essential for every exerciser to secure medical clearance, including a stress electrocardiogram, before beginning an exercise program. Beginning a program isn't recommended for anyone over age sixty *unless* adequate cardiovascular screening, including a stress ECG, has been accomplished and there are no signs or symptoms of heart disease. If you do begin at this age, you should have a thorough exam every two years.

Swimming Exercise Programs (To 49 years)

Beginner

Week	Distance (yards)	Time Goal (minutes)	Frequency/Week (sessions)
1	300	12:00	4
2	400	14:00	4
3	600	18:00	4
4	800	21:30	4
5	900	25:00	4
6	1000	27:30	4
7	1100	30:30	4
8	1200	33:15	4
9	1300	36:00	3

Week	Distance (yards)	Time Goal (minutes)	Frequency/Week (sessions)
10	1400	38:00	3
11	1500	41:30	3
12	1600	45:00	3

Recreational

(swimmers wishing to improve speed and/or endurance)

Week	Distance (yards)	Time Goal (minutes)	Frequency/Week (sessions)
1	400	10:00	4
2	500	12:30	4
3	600	15:00	4
4	700	17:30	4
5	800	20:00	4
6	900	22:30	4
7	1000	25:00	4
8	1200	30:00	3
9	1400	35:00	3
10	1600	40:00	3

Elite

(competitive swimmers wanting to improve speed and/or endurance)

Week	Distance (yards)	Time Goal (minutes)	Frequency/Week (sessions)
1	500 (x3)	9:00 5:00 rest	5
2	500 (x3)	8:00 5:00 rest	5
3	600 (x3)	10:00 5:00 rest	5
4	800	13:00	5
5	1000	16:30	5
6	750 (x2)	<12:30 5:00 rest	2
	1000	16:00	2
7	1200	19:30	4
8	400	6:15 4:00 rest	2
	1200	19:00	2
9	1400	23:00	4
10	1600	26:00	2
	800 (x2)	12:00 5:00 rest	2
11	1800	29:30	4

Swimming Exercise Programs (To 49 years)—Cont'd
Elite

Week	Distance (yards)	Time Goal (minutes)	Frequency/Week (sessions)
12	2000	33:00	1
	200 (x4)	2:45 2:00 rest	2
	1600	25:00	2

< means less than

Swimming Exercise Programs (50–59 years)
Beginner

Week	Distance (yards)	Time Goal (minutes)	Frequency/Week (sessions)
1	200	8:30	4
2	300	12:00	4
3	400	14:00	4
4	500	16:00	4
5	600	18:00	4
6	700	21:00	4
7	800	24:30	4
8	900	27:30	4
9	1000	30:00	4
10	1100	33:30	4
11	1200	36:30	3
12	1300	39:30	3
13	1400	42:00	3
14	1500	46:00	3

Recreational
(swimmers wishing to improve speed and/or endurance)

Week	Distance (yards)	Time Goal (minutes)	Frequency/Week (sessions)
1	400	11:00	4
2	500	13:30	4
3	600	16:00	4
4	700	18:30	4
5	800	21:00	4
6	900	23:30	4
7	1000	26:00	4

Week	Distance (yards)	Time Goal (minutes)	Frequency/Week (sessions)
8	1200	31:00	3
9	1400	36:00	3
10	1600	41:00	3

Elite

(competitive swimmer wanting to improve speed and/or endurance)

Week	Distance (yards)	Time Goal (minutes)	Frequency/Week (sessions)
1	400 (x2)	8:00 5:00 rest	5
2	500 (x2)	10:00 5:00 rest	5
3	500 (x3)	9:00 5:00 rest	5
4	600 (x2)	11:00 5:00 rest	5
5	800	15:00	5
6	1000	19:00	5
7	1000	18:00	2
	400 (x3)	6:30 4:00 rest	2
8	1200	22:00	4
9	1400	26:00	2
	400 (x3)	6:15 4:00 rest	2
10	1600	30:00	1
	300 (x4)	5:00 3:00 rest	2
	1000	18:00	1
11	1800	30:00	4
12	2000	34:00	1
	200 (x4)	3:00	2
	1500	26:00	2

Swimming Exercise Programs (60–69 years)
Beginner

Week	Distance (yards)	Time Goal (minutes)	Frequency/Week (sessions)
1	200	9:00	4
2	200	8:00	4
3	300	12:30	4
4	300	12:00	4

Swimming Exercise Programs (60–69 years)—Cont'd
Beginner

Week	Distance (yards)	Time Goal (minutes)	Frequency/Week (sessions)
5	400	14:00	4
6	500	16:00	4
7	600	19:00	4
8	700	22:00	4
9	800	25:00	4
10	900	28:00	4
11	1000	31:00	4
12	1100	34:00	3
13	1200	37:00	3
14	1300	40:00	3
15	1400	43:00	3

Recreational
(swimmers who wish to improve speed and/or endurance)

Week	Distance (yards)	Time Goal (minutes)	Frequency/Week (sessions)
1	300	9:30	4
2	400	12:00	4
3	500	14:30	4
4	600	17:00	4
5	700	19:30	4
6	800	22:00	4
7	900	24:30	4
8	1000	27:00	3
9	1200	32:00	3
10	1400	37:00	3

Elite
(competitive swimmers who want to improve speed and/or endurance)

Week	Distance (yards)	Time Goal (minutes)	Frequency/Week (sessions)
1	300 (x2)	7:30 5:00 rest	5
2	400 (x2)	9:00 5:00 rest	5
3	500 (x2)	11:00 5:00 rest	5

Week	Distance (yards)	Time Goal (minutes)		Frequency/Week (sessions)
4	600 (x2)	13:00	5:00 rest	5
5	700	15:00	5:00 rest	4
	500	10:00		4
6	800	17:00		4
7	1000	20:00		3
	500 (x2)	9:30	5:00 rest	2
8	1100	22:00		4
9	1200	24:00		2
10	1300	26:00		4
11	1400	28:00		4
12	1500	30:00		2
	300 (x4)	5:30	3:00 rest	2
	1600	32:00		1

Swimming Exercise Programs (70+ years)
Beginner

Week	Distance (yards)	Time Goal (minutes)	Frequency/Week (sessions)
1	100	5:00	4
2	150	7:30	4
3	200	9:00	4
4	250	12:00	4
5	300	14:00	4
6	400	16:30	4
7	500	16:30	4
8	600	20:00	4
9	700	23:00	4
10	800	26:30	4
11	900	30:00	4
12	1000	33:20	4
13	1100	36:40	4
14	1200	39:30	3
15	1300	43:30	3
16	1400	46:30	3
17	1500	50:00	3

Recreational

(swimmers who wish to improve speed and/or endurance)

Week	Distance (yards)	Time Goal (minutes)	Frequency/Week (sessions)
1	200	8:00	4
2	250	9:00	4
3	300	10:00	4
4	350	11:30	4
5	400	13:00	4
6	450	15:00	4
7	500	16:30	4
8	600	19:00	4
9	700	16:30	4
10	800	24:00	4
11	900	26:30	4
12	1000	29:00	4

Note: Elite program not recommended for this age group.

GUIDE TO PROGRAMS FOR MISCELLANEOUS ENDURANCE ACTIVITIES (INCLUDING AEROBIC DANCING, STEP AEROBICS, STAIR CLIMBING, STATIONARY RUNNING, ROPE SKIPPING, ROWING MACHINES, AND CROSS-COUNTRY SKI SIMULATORS)

1. Do a three- to five-minute warm-up of calisthenics or slow movements that mimic your chosen exercise. Don't worry too much about your performance at the beginning of each week, but by the end of the week, attempt to reach the stated goal. If you can't achieve the final goal, repeat the week.

2. Always cool down with slow movements that mimic the exercise for five minutes after completing the measured distance.

3. The RPE column represents the Rate of Perceived Exertion in more precise numerical terms, according to the Borg scale that was discussed previously. I've included a wider range of perceived exertion categories here because some of these miscellaneous activities may place unusual demands on muscles that haven't been used in a while. To avoid injury or other discomfort, it's always best to start at a very low level of intensity when you're engaging in activities that feel strange to your body. Then, if you like, you can work up to a harder workout when your muscles are better conditioned and your skill at the activity has improved.

4. The ten to twelve RPE range, as indicated on the charts, indicates a perceived effort of "very light" to "fairly light" for those at the very beginning of one of their programs. The thirteen to fourteen range is where you'll be after a couple of weeks, when you feel your exertion has become

"somewhat hard." The fifteen to sixteen category involves a Rate of Perceived Exertion of "hard, or heavy" exercise. Finally, the seventeen to eighteen rating—which I would *not* recommend for anyone except those training to reach the very highest level of conditioning—is a perceived effort of "*very hard,*" where you feel you can "still go on, but have to push."

5. At the end of seven weeks, the duration and intensity of the activity will be sufficient to provide adequate conditioning. Those who want to get in even better shape may progress to the twelfth week.

6. All the programs can be used by men or women.

7. It's essential for every exerciser to secure medical clearance, including a stress electrocardiogram, before beginning an exercise program. Beginning a program isn't recommended for anyone over age sixty *unless* adequate cardiovascular screening, including a stress ECG, has been accomplished and there are no signs or symptoms of heart disease. If you do begin at this age, you should have a thorough exam every two years.

Miscellaneous Endurance Exercise Program

Age (in years)

Week	RPE	40–49	50–59	60–69	70+	Frequency/Week (sessions)
1	**B** 10–12	18:00	15:00	12:30	10:00	4–5
2	**E** 10–12	20:00	16:00	14:00	11:00	4–5
3	**G** 10–12	22:00	18:00	16:00	12:00	4–5
4	**I** 10–12	24:00	20:00	18:00	14:00	4–5
5	**N** 13–14	26:00	22:00	20:00	16:00	4–5
6	**N** 13–14	28:00	24:00	22:00	18:00	4–5
7	**E** 13–14 **R**	30:00	25:00	25:00	20:00	4–5
8	**A** 15–16	32:00	28:00	25:00	22:00	4–5
9	**D** 15–16	34:00	30:00	28:00	24:00	4–5
10	**V** 15–16	36:00	33:00	30:00	26:00	4–5
11	**A** 17–18	40:00	36:00	32:00	28:00	4–5
12	**N** 17–18 **C** **E** **D**	45:00	40:00	35:00	30:00	4–5

8

BY REASON OF STRENGTH

Strength is an extremely important factor for both spiritual and physical fitness. King David, in his inspiring eighteenth psalm, recognized the connection between the spiritual and physical when he wrote: "It is God who arms me with strength, / And makes my way perfect. / He makes my feet like the feet of deer, / And sets me on my high places."

Yet for some reason, David lacked the strength to live more than seventy years, and in fact, during his last days, he lay incapacitated in bed. Perhaps some of the accumulated errors of his ways, such as committing adultery with Bathsheba and arranging for the death of her husband, Uriah, caught up with him. Or maybe he just didn't take care of himself physically. In any event, he fell short of the fourscore years that Psalm 90 tells us can be achieved "by reason of strength."

Are there any lessons we can learn from King David's experience? Certainly, if we remain close to God through obedience, prayer, and other spiritual disciplines, his strength will flow into us. At the same time, it's incumbent on us to take care of our bodies, including our muscles.

We have already seen in chapter 4 that scientific studies, including groundbreaking research at Tufts University, have revealed that even people in their nineties can achieve significant improvement in their muscular strength and tone with exercise. Endurance activities, such as walking or jogging, just aren't enough to give your body the all-around muscular conditioning it needs. What's required, in addition to endurance exercise, is a strength program involving calisthenics, weights, or some similar muscle-building activity. That's what a longtime jogger named Charlie discovered when he was confronted with some physical challenges he couldn't quite handle.

What Can Strength Training Do That Endurance Training Can't?

Charlie, a fifty-two-year-old attorney from the Midwest, had been jogging for nearly ten years, and he consistently scored in the "superior" category on endurance-keyed treadmill stress tests. He had become a little smug because it seemed he was in much better aerobic shape than almost all his friends his age. But he was in for a rude surprise when he went for testing at a special fitness evaluation and training center that had just opened in his area.

There had been some earlier signals that all might not be well with his body. On one vacation trip with his family, he went out for an extended bicycle ride for the first time in more than twenty years. By the time he returned, his hands, wrists, and shoulders were cramping painfully from holding and leaning over the handlebars. Also, his thighs were so sore the next morning he could hardly get out of bed. A few weeks later, when he was doing some repair work around his home, he strained his wrist while positioning a heavy board on a workbench.

The full picture of Charlie's muscle problems emerged at the fitness center. Strength testing showed that his arm strength and chest strength were only in the thirtieth percentile for his age group. Also, his thigh muscles and his hamstring muscles (on the back of the thighs) were in the fortieth percentile. His abdominal muscles registered in only the forty-fifth percentile.

The physiologist supervising Charlie's tests recommended a series of exercises to strengthen his weak muscles, and he was shocked enough by the test results to embark immediately on the corrective program. The physiologist motivated him further by issuing this warning:

"It's essential at your age to get your muscles in shape. If you don't, you'll lose significant amounts of muscle every year—maybe one to two percent of your muscle mass annually. This means that by the time you get into your sixties, and certainly your seventies, your heart and endurance could be in good shape from your running, but you could be vulnerable to serious injury from weak muscles. This might force you to stop running, and a possible end result is that you could easily become at least partially incapacitated, maybe for years."

That prospect disturbed Charlie deeply, not just because he might lose physical functioning, but because such incapacity would jeopardize the plans he had been laying for retirement. He wanted to leave his law firm by the time he was sixty and launch a second career as a foreign missionary. He and his wife had been saving diligently toward this end so that they could cover their own expenses in some form of lay ministry overseas. But Charlie now realized that this dream might become impossible unless he did something to stop his physical deterioration.

So he began a rather simple but highly effective three-times-per-week strength training program that combined calisthenics and light weight work. Although he varied the exercises he did, the mainstay of his regimen involved this routine:

- push-ups and bench presses with barbells for the arms, shoulders, and chest
- sit-ups for his abdominal muscles
- for his upper legs, lunges (long, forward steps with one leg) while holding a light dumbbell in each hand

Within a month, Charlie noticed significant improvement in the strength and muscle definition of those parts of his body he was exercising. When he returned to the fitness center for an evaluation six months later, he increased his test performance by more than 20 percent in all of the strength categories!

Charlie's story—and his achievement—aren't unusual. *Most* people over thirty have started to lose significant amounts of muscle strength over what they possessed in their late teens and early twenties. And the situation gets worse the older you get. Unfortunately, the large majority of men and women never catch on to what is happening to their bodies until they begin to lose physical function, and by then, it may be too late to do anything about it.

It's easy to be fooled if you're an endurance athlete like Charlie because one part of your body, your cardiovascular system, may be in great shape. It's also easy to be fooled if you've managed to stay about the same weight at age forty or fifty as you were at age twenty. But don't allow the wool to be pulled over your eyes! It's almost certain that if you haven't been exercising regularly, your percent of body fat will have gone up, even though your weight has remained the same. In other words, your body will have "redistributed" itself, with more fat and less muscle—a condition that greatly increases your risk of disease, injury, and eventual loss of physical function.

Yet, like Charlie, you don't have to resign yourself to a steady loss of muscle tissue or some degree of eventual incapacity. You can do something to recapture any loss of strength by embarking on one of the strength programs in this chapter.

The Muscular Strength Programs

The following strength exercises have been divided into three types of activity: calisthenics, light circuit, weight training, and aqua-aerobics training. Each type of activity contains exercises designed to condition three basic muscle groups:

Muscle Group #1: arms, shoulders, and chest
Muscle Group #2: abdomen and trunk
Muscle Group #3: legs and lower back

In designing your own strength program, you should choose *at least one* of the exercises listed for each of these muscle groups. As you grow stronger, you'll probably find you want to add additional exercises for each muscle group.

You have a choice. If you like, you can alternate between two (or more) of the four exercise classifications. For example, you might choose to exercise the first two muscle groups with calisthenics (push-ups, chin-ups, and sit-ups), and the last group with handweights (lunges and calf raises). To assist you in making your choices, I've noted in the exercise descriptions the specific muscle groups that benefit from the different exercises.

Whichever variation you choose, you should do a minimum of twenty minutes of strength exercises, three times a week. It will usually take you four to six weeks to reach the goals indicated in the exercises.

The Calisthenics Programs

A GUIDE TO THE PROGRAMS

1. Get clearance from your doctor, especially if you have a medical problem, such as heart disease, arthritis, or hypertension.

2. Always warm up by spending three to five minutes doing light stretching or running in place.

3. Work out all three main muscle groups. Don't fall into the trap of focusing on only one part of the body. The exercises should be done in the order listed, though it's acceptable to skip an occasional exercise if you run out of time or lack energy on a given day. But remember, at least one exercise must be done for each of the three muscle groups.

4. Always wait a day between strength workouts.

5. Pay close attention to proper breathing: Inhale as you start each movement, and exhale as you complete the movement. Don't hold your breath during the exercises.

6. Each exercise should be performed with a complete range of motion, both to get the maximum strength benefit and to promote stretching and flexibility.

7. To improve your strength, you'll eventually want to do two sets of each exercise. A "set" refers to a duplication of an exercise in a short period of time. In other words, to do two sets of push-ups, you might perform twenty repetitions; then you'd rest for fifteen to sixty seconds; finally, you'd perform another twenty repetitions. Strength training depends on the "over-

load principle"—you build strength and power by increasing the work your muscles must do.

Calisthenics for Muscle Group #1: Arms, Shoulders, and Chest

MODIFIED PUSH-UPS

Get down on the floor with your body supported only by hands and knees. Your hands should be about shoulder-width apart and placed just below your head, with fingers pointed forward. Straighten your spine so that your back is parallel to the floor.

Keeping your back straight, lower your body toward the floor until your chin touches. Then push your body up to the starting position. This movement constitutes one repetition.

This exercise strengthens the chest, back of the upper arms, and shoulders.

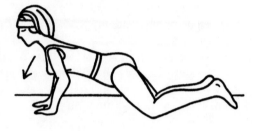

Goals for Different Age Groups (These are the number of repetitions to be performed in one set of the exercise, without interruption. Begin with the lowest number of repetitions and increase gradually to the highest number over a six-week period. An additional set may be added as strength and endurance increase.)

Age (in years)	*Repetitions in one set*
To 49	25–40
50–59	20–35
60–69	15–30
70+	10–25

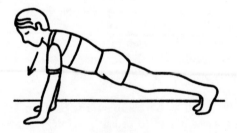

STANDARD PUSH-UPS

Lie flat on your stomach on the floor. Place your hands flat on the floor next to your chest. Push straight up until your arms and elbows are straight. Support your body only with your hands and toes. Keep your back straight. Lower your body back to the starting position. This movement constitutes one repetition.

This exercise strengthens the chest, back of the upper arms, and shoulders.

Goals for Different Age Groups (These are the number of repetitions to be performed in one set of the exercise, without interruption. Begin with the lowest number of repetitions and increase gradually to the highest number over a six-week period. An additional set may be added as strength and endurance increase.)

Age (in years)	Repetitions in one set
To 49	10–30
50–59	10–25
60–69	5–20
70+	5–10

ARM LIFTS

Begin in the sitting position, with your upper body inclined slightly backward, hands flat on the floor behind your buttocks, and arms and elbows straight.

Bring your hips off the floor, while keeping your head back and body straight. Your body should be supported entirely by the hands and heels. Hold this position for one to three seconds, and then drop your hips back to the floor. This movement constitutes one repetition.

This exercise benefits the back of the arms and the shoulders.

Goals for Different Age Groups (These are the number of repetitions to be performed in one set of the exercise, without interruption. Begin with the lowest number of repetitions and increase gradually to the highest number over a six-week period. Additional sets, up to a total of three sets, may be added as strength and endurance increase.)

Age (in years)	Repetitions in one set
To 49	15–30
50–59	10–25
60–69	10–20
70+	5–10

PULL-UPS

Using an overhand grip, grasp a horizontal chin-up bar that is positioned above your head. Begin the exercise in a hanging position, with your arms straight and your feet off the floor. Pull up until your chin is above the bar. Return to the hanging position. This movement constitutes one repetition. (Caution: Breathe while you perform this exercise—don't hold your breath.)

This exercise strengthens the biceps, wrists, and shoulders.

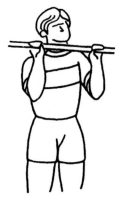

Goals for Different Age Groups (These are the number of repetitions to be performed in one set of the exercise, without interruption. Begin with the lowest number of repetitions and increase gradually to the highest number over a six-week period. An additional set may be added as strength and endurance increase.)

Age (in years)	Repetitions in one set
To 49	2–15
50–59	2–12
60–69	2–10
70+	1–5

NEGATIVE PULL-UPS

(For those who have difficulty performing a regular pull-up.) Stand in the upright position on a stool, which allows you to position your chin above the horizontal bar. Place your hands on the bar so that the palms are turned inward, toward your face.

Lift your feet off the stool and suspend your body only with your arms and hands. Lower your body slowly until your arms are straight, with your feet lifted off the stool. Stand on the stool, and assume your original upright position. This movement constitutes one repetition.

This exercise strengthens the biceps, wrists, and shoulders.

Goals for Different Age Groups (These are the number of repetitions to be performed in one set of the exercise, without interruption. Begin with the lowest number of repetitions and increase gradually to the highest number over a six-week period. An additional set may be added as strength and endurance increase.)

Age (in years)	Repetitions in one set
To 49	5–15
50–59	5–12
60–69	3–10
70+	2–5

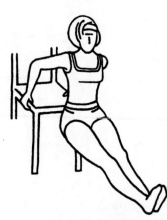

SEAT DROP

Use a sturdy chair or other solid, raised surface. Support your body with your hands planted on the top of the chair, with your arms and legs fully extended. Your body weight should be on your heels and hands. Lower your body until your buttocks touch the floor. Straighten your arms and return your body to the original position. This movement constitutes one repetition.

This exercise strengthens the back of the upper arms, the shoulders, and the stomach.

Goals for Different Age Groups (These are the number of repetitions to be performed in one set of the exercise, without interruption. Begin with the lowest number of repetitions and increase gradually to the highest

number over a six-week period. An additional set may be added as strength and endurance increase.)

Age (in years)	Repetitions in one set
To 49	5–12
50–59	4–10
60–69	3–10
70+	2–8

Calisthenics for Muscle Group #2: Abdomen and Trunk

MODIFIED SIT-UPS

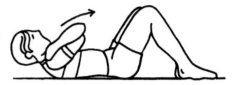

Lie flat on your back on the floor, with knees off the floor at a forty-five-degree angle and feet flat on the floor. Your arms should be crossed across your chest.

Curl up your upper body toward your knees, so that your shoulders are off the ground. Hold this position for one count and then slowly lower your upper body down to the starting position. This movement constitutes one repetition.

This exercise strengthens the abdominal muscles.

Goals for Different Age Groups (These are the number of repetitions to be performed in one set of the exercise, without interruption. Begin with the lowest number of repetitions and increase gradually to the highest number over a six-week period. An additional set may be added as strength and endurance increase.)

Age (in years)	Repetitions in one set
To 49	10–20
50–59	8–15
60–69	6–12
70+	5–10

SIDE-REACH CRUNCHES

Lie flat on your back on the floor, with knees off the floor at a forty-five-degree angle and feet flat on the floor. Your arms should be held straight down along the floor, next to your body.

Move your chin up to your chest, and curl up no more than forty-five degrees off the floor. Extend your right hand down along the side of your trunk and reach toward your right heel. Return to the starting position. This movement constitutes one repetition. For the next repetition, reach your left hand down along the side of your trunk toward your left heel.

This exercise strengthens the abdominal and side muscles.

Goals for Different Age Groups (These are the number of repetitions to be performed in one set of the exercise, without interruption. Begin with the lowest number of repetitions and increase gradually to the highest

number over a six-week period. An additional set may be added as strength and endurance increase.)

Age (in years)	Repetitions in one set
To 49	10–20
50–59	8–15
60–69	6–12
70+	5–10

FULL SIT-UPS

Lie flat on your back on the floor, with knees off the floor at a forty-five-degree angle and feet flat on the floor. Your arms should be crossed across your chest.

Raise your upper body to a sitting position. Lower your upper body to the starting position. This movement constitutes one repetition.

This exercise strengthens the abdominal muscles.

Goals for Different Age Groups (These are the number of repetitions to be performed in one set of the exercise, without interruption. Begin with the lowest number of repetitions and increase gradually to the highest number over a six-week period. An additional set may be added as strength and endurance increase.)

Age (in years)	Repetitions in one set
To 49	25–50
50–59	22–45
60–69	20–40
70+	15–30

HIP CURLS

Lie on the floor with fingers locked behind your head. Either keep your head on the floor throughout, or keep it supported up with your chin on your chest. Knees are bent and squeezed together, with the lower legs relaxed.

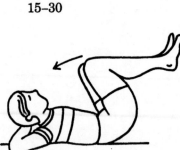

Contract your lower abdominal area to curl your hips off the ground about five inches, so that your knees approach your chest. Don't expect to curl up very high.

Slowly round your hips back down to the ground. Don't whip your legs to help you get your hips up. This movement constitutes one repetition.

This exercise strengthens the lower abdominal muscles, the upper thighs, and the hips.

Goals for Different Age Groups (These are the number of repetitions to be performed in one set of the exercise, without interruption. Begin with the lowest number of repetitions and increase gradually to the highest

number over a six-week period. An additional set may be added as strength and endurance increase.)

Age (in years)	Repetitions in one set
To 49	8–12
50–59	5–10
60–69	Not recommended
70+	Not recommended

Calisthenics for Muscle Group #3: Legs and Lower Back

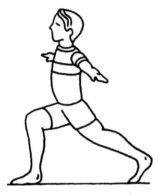

FORWARD LUNGE

Stand with your feet shoulder-width apart and your hands on your hips or your arms extended out to the side as though you were about to "flap your wings." Take a long step forward with your left foot. Your left leg should be bent at the knee and your right leg extended straight out to the rear. Keep your back straight, and lower your hips as far as possible toward the floor. Return to the starting position. This movement constitutes one repetition. For the second repetition, step forward with your right foot.

Caution: Do not let the knee of the forward, thrusting leg move beyond the forward foot.

This exercise strengthens the thigh muscles and the lower back.

Goals for Different Age Groups (These are the number of repetitions to be performed in one set of the exercise, without interruption. Begin with the lowest number of repetitions and increase gradually to the highest number over a six-week period. An additional set may be added as strength and endurance increase.)

Age (in years)	Repetitions in one set
To 49	10–20
50–59	8–18
60–69	6–15
70+	5–10

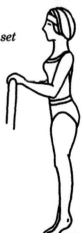

CALF RAISES

Standing erect, raise your body up on your toes as high as possible. Return to the standing position. If necessary, balance yourself by placing your hand against a wall or railing. This movement constitutes one repetition. For more challenging resistance, place a one- or two-inch block of wood, or other raised surface, under your toes.

This exercise strengthens the calf muscles.

Goals for Different Age Groups (These are the number of repetitions to be performed in one set of the exercise, without interruption. Begin with the lowest number of repetitions and increase gradually to the highest number over a six-week period. An additional set may be added as strength and endurance increase.)

Age (in years)	Repetitions in one set
To 49	10–30
50–59	10–25
60–69	8–20
70+	5–15

SCISSOR LEG LIFTS

Lie on your left side, with your left leg straight down in line with your body. Bend your right knee, and place your right foot behind the knee of your left leg.

Supporting yourself with your hands and elbows, raise your right leg straight up. Return your right leg to the starting position. This movement constitutes one repetition.

Repeat the exercise for the required number of repetitions indicated below. Then, repeat the exercise for the right side.

This exercise strengthens the outer thighs and hips.

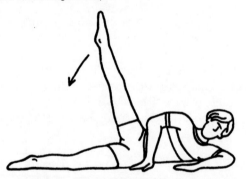

Goals for Different Age Groups (These are the number of repetitions to be performed in one set of the exercise, without interruption. Begin with the lowest number of repetitions and increase gradually to the highest number over a six-week period. An additional set may be added as strength and endurance increase.)

Age (in years)	Repetitions in one set
To 49	10–30
50–59	10–25
60–69	8–20
70+	5–15

REAR LEG LIFTS

Kneel with your elbows and knees on the floor in a "baby crawl" position. Keeping your left leg bent and on the floor, slowly extend your right leg straight back and raise it with your knee bent toward the ceiling as far as you can. Return your right leg to the starting position. This movement constitutes one repetition. Repeat until you've finished the required number of repetitions indicated below. Then, go through the same movements with your left leg.

This exercise strengthens the muscles in the back of the legs, the lower back, and the buttocks.

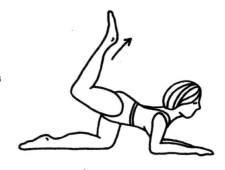

Goals for Different Age Groups (These are the number of repetitions to be performed in one set of the exercise, without interruption. Begin with the lowest number of repetitions and increase gradually to the highest number over a six-week period. An additional set may be added as strength and endurance increase.)

Age (in years)	Repetitions in one set
To 49	15–30
50–59	15–25
60–69	10–20
70+	5–15

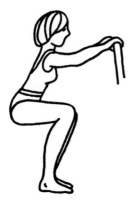

HALF SQUATS

Stand straight while holding onto a bar, the back of a chair, or some other solid object. Bend your knees until your thighs are almost at right angles to your lower legs. Hold this position for one second, and return to the standing position. This movement constitutes one repetition.

Caution: Do not squat down any farther than this or you may injure your knee.

This exercise strengthens the front of the thighs.

Goals for Different Age Groups (These are the number of repetitions to be performed in one set of the exercise, without interruption. Begin with the lowest number of repetitions and increase gradually to the highest number over a six-week period. An additional set may be added as strength and endurance increase.)

Age (in years)	Repetitions in one set
To 49	15–30
50–59	15–25
60–69	8–20
70+	5–15

Light Weight Circuit Training Program

A GUIDE TO THE CIRCUIT TRAINING PROGRAMS

1. Get clearance from your doctor, especially if you have a medical problem, such as heart disease, arthritis, or hypertension.

2. Always warm up by spending three to five minutes doing light stretching or running in place.

3. Work out all three main muscle groups. Don't fall into the trap of focusing on only one part of the body. The exercises should be done in the order listed, though it's acceptable to skip an occasional exercise if you run out of time or lack energy on a given day. But remember, at least one exercise must be done for each of the three muscle groups.

4. Women who are just beginning these exercises should use weights that are one-and-a-half to three pounds each. The beginning weight for men should be three to five pounds. As fitness improves, women can work up to five pound dumbbells. Men may increase their weight to ten pounds.

5. In using weights, begin at a level of resistance that allows you to perform at least eight consecutive repetitions of the exercise. This minimum number of repetitions has been found to be ideal for developing a combination of strength and muscle stamina.

6. The recommended exercises should be performed on three separate days each week, preferably with at least one day of rest in between exercise days.

7. Pay close attention to proper breathing: Inhale as you start the movement, and exhale as you complete the movement. Never hold your breath during an exercise.

8. Maintain good posture at all times during the exercises.

9. Each exercise should be performed with a complete, steady range of motion, both to get the maximum strength benefit and to promote stretching and flexibility. There should be no jerky movements.

10. For the first week or two, perform only one set of the suggested repetitions of each exercise.

11. To improve your strength, you'll eventually want to do two sets of an exercise, with fifteen to sixty seconds of rest between sets. A "set" refers to a duplication of repetitions of an exercise within a short period of time. In other words, to do two sets of a bench press, you might perform twelve repetitions; then you'd rest for up to one minute; finally, you'd perform another

twelve repetitions. Strength training depends on the "overload principle"—you build strength and power by increasing the work your muscles must do.

Light Weight Training for Muscle Group #1: Arms, Shoulders, and Chest

LYING BENCH PRESS

Lie flat on a bench, with knees bent and feet flat. Hold the dumbbells against your upper chest in each hand, shoulder-width apart, with palms facing toward your feet.

Push the dumbbells straight up and return to the starting position. This movement constitutes one repetition.

This exercise strengthens the chest muscles and the back of the upper arms.

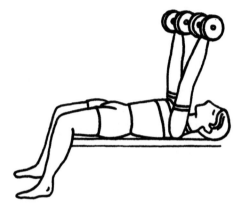

Goals for Different Age Groups (These are the number of repetitions to be performed in one set of the exercise, without interruption. Begin with the lowest number of repetitions and increase gradually to the highest number over a six-week period. An additional set may be added as strength and endurance increase.)

Age (in years)	Repetitions in one set
To 49	10–20
50–59	8–18
60–69	8–16
70+	6–12

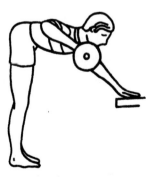

BENT-OVER ROWING

Stand bending over at the waist, with one hand on the bench for balance. Hold one dumbbell in your free hand, with your arm fully extended. Pull the dumbbell up to your shoulder, then lower the dumbbell to the starting position. This movement represents one repetition. When the required repetitions and sets are completed with one arm, repeat with your other arm.

This exercise strengthens the back and the biceps.

Goals for Different Age Groups (These are the number of repetitions to be performed in one set of the exercise, without interruption. Begin with

the lowest number of repetitions and increase gradually to the highest number over a six-week period. An additional set may be added as strength and endurance increase.)

Age (in years)	Repetitions in one set
To 49	10–20
50–59	8–18
60–69	8–16
70+	6–12

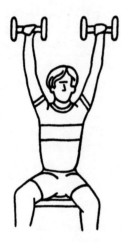

SEATED OVERHEAD PRESS

Sit on a bench with your back supported against a back rest. Hold a dumbbell in each hand against the chest, with arms bent and palms facing forward.

Push the dumbbells straight up until your arms are fully extended. Lower slowly to the starting position. The movement constitutes one repetition.

This exercise strengthens the shoulders, and the back of the upper arms.

Goals for Different Age Groups (These are the number of repetitions to be performed in one set of the exercise, without interruption. Begin with the lowest number of repetitions and increase gradually to the highest number over a six-week period. An additional set may be added as strength and endurance increase.)

Age (in years)	Repetitions in one set
To 49	10–20
50–59	8–18
60–69	8–16
70+	6–12

ARM CIRCLES

Stand erect with feet together and arms horizontal to sides. Grasping a light weight in each hand, commence a rapid, small circle action toward the rear and then back toward the front. Keep your arms and wrists locked throughout. One complete circular motion constitutes one repetition.

This exercise strengthens the shoulders and upper arms.

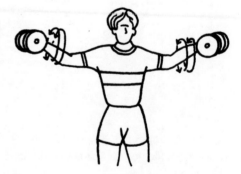

Goals for Different Age Groups (These are the number of repetitions to be performed in one set of the exercise, without interruption. Begin with the lowest number of repetitions and increase gradually to the highest number over a six-week period. An additional set may be added as strength and endurance increase.)

Age (in years)	Repetitions in one set
To 49	20–30
50–59	18–28
60–69	15–25
70+	10–20

SIDE ARM RAISES

Stand erect, with your feet shoulder-width apart and your arms at your sides. Holding a light weight in each hand and keeping your arms straight, raise your arms to an extended position above your head. Lower slowly. This movement constitutes one repetition.

This exercise strengthens the shoulders and upper arms.

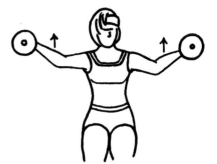

Goals for Different Age Groups (These are the number of repetitions to be performed in one set of the exercise, without interruption. Begin with the lowest number of repetitions and increase gradually to the highest number over a six-week period. An additional set may be added as strength and endurance increase.)

Age (in years)	Repetitions in one set
To 49	10–20
50–59	8–18
60–69	8–15
70+	5–10

Light Weight Training for Muscle Group #2: Abdomen and Trunk

SEATED SIDE BENDS

Sit upright in a chair, with your legs open and your feet about two to three feet apart. Grasp your dumbbells, and raise your arms straight out to the sides at shoulder height, parallel to the floor. Keep your arms and back straight. Do not lean forward.

Bend sideways at the waist to the right, and move the dumbbell in your right hand toward the floor on your right side, though you probably won't be able to touch the floor. Hold this position for five seconds and relax. Return to

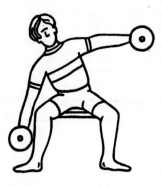

the starting position and repeat the same movement to your left side. The complete movements to both sides constitute one repetition.

This exercise strengthens the muscles on the side of the abdomen.

Goals for Different Age Groups (These are the number of repetitions to be performed in one set of the exercise, without interruption. Begin with the lowest number of repetitions and increase gradually to the highest number over a six-week period. An additional set may be added as strength and endurance increase.)

Age (in years)	Repetitions in one set
To 49	10–20
50–59	8–18
60–69	8–15
70+	5–10

WEIGHTED SIT-UPS

Lie flat on your back, and bend your legs at a forty-five degree angle. Your feet should be flat on the floor and may be secured, such as by having a partner hold them against the floor. Grasp a dumbbell in each hand, and place your arms across your chest. Slowly lift your body halfway to the vertical position, then slowly move back to the starting position. This movement constitutes one repetition.

This exercise strengthens the abdominal muscles.

Goals for Different Age Groups (These are the number of repetitions to be performed in one set of the exercise, without interruption. Begin with the lowest number of repetitions and increase gradually to the highest number over a six-week period. An additional set may be added as strength and endurance increase.)

Age (in years)	Repetitions in one set
To 49	10–25
50–59	10–20
60–69	8–16
70+	5–10

Light Weight Training for Muscle Group #3: Legs and Lower Back

FORWARD DUMBBELL LUNGES

Stand with your feet shoulder-width apart, arms hanging at your sides with a dumbbell in each hand. Take a long step forward with your left foot, and bend your left knee, but not beyond a ninety-degree angle. Your right leg should remain extended straight out to the rear. Keep your back straight. Return to the starting position. This movement constitutes one repetition. For the second repetition, step forward with your right foot.

Caution: Do not let the knee of the forward, thrusting leg move beyond the foot.

This exercise strengthens the front of the thighs and the lower back.

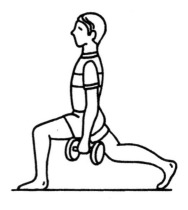

Goals for Different Age Groups (These are the number of repetitions to be performed in one set of the exercise, without interruption. Begin with the lowest number of repetitions and increase gradually to the highest number over a six-week period. An additional set may be added as strength and endurance increase.)

Age (in years)	*Repetitions in one set*
To 49	8–15
50–59	6–12
60–69	6–12
70+	5–10

CALF RAISES WITH DUMBBELLS

Grasp a dumbbell in each hand and stand straight, with arms hanging down at your sides. Raise your body up on your toes as high as possible. Return to the standing position by lowering your heels to the floor. This movement constitutes one repetition.

Goals for Different Age Groups (These are the number of repetitions to be performed in one set of the exercise, without interruption. Begin with the lowest number of repetitions and increase gradually to the highest number over a six-week period. An additional set may be added as strength and endurance increase.)

Age (in years)	*Repetitions in one set*
To 49	10–20
50–59	8–18
60–69	8–18
70+	6–12

The Aqua-Aerobics Programs

A GUIDE TO THE AQUA-AEROBICS PROGRAM

1. Get clearance from your doctor, especially if you have a medical problem, such as heart disease, arthritis, or hypertension.

2. Always warm up by spending three to five minutes doing light calisthenics or light swimming.

3. Work out all three main muscle groups. Don't fall into the trap of focusing on only one part of the body. The exercises should be done in the order listed, though it's acceptable to skip an occasional exercise if you run out of time or lack energy on a given day. But remember, at least one exercise must be done for each of the three muscle groups.

4. Always leave a day between strength workouts.

5. Pay close attention to proper breathing: Inhale as you start the movement, and exhale as you complete the movement. Don't hold your breath during the exercises.

6. Each exercise should be performed with a complete range of motion, both to get the maximum strength benefit and to promote stretching and flexibility.

7. To improve your strength, you'll eventually want to do two to three sets of an exercise. A "set" refers to a duplication of an exercise in a short period of time. In other words, to do two sets of the circular arm exercise, you might perform twelve repetitions; then you'd rest for fifteen to sixty seconds; and finally, you'd perform another twelve repetitions. Strength training depends on the "overload principle"—you build strength and power by increasing the work your muscles must do.

Aqua-Aerobics for Muscle Group #1: Arms, Shoulders, and Chest

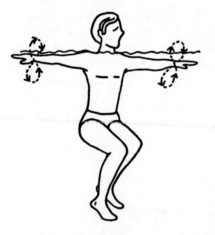

ARM CIRCLES

Enter water almost shoulder high, put your right foot in front of the left, and bend both knees slightly so that your shoulders and arms are beneath the surface. Hold your arms straight out to the sides, with palms facing down.

Moving both your arms together, trace figure eights with your hands in the water. Keep your fingers together and your elbows and arms straight to increase the resistance. Tracing one figure eight constitutes one repetition.

This exercise benefits the shoulders, chest, and upper arms.

Goals for Different Age Groups (These are the number of repetitions to be performed in one set of the exercise, without interruption. Begin with

the lowest number of repetitions and increase gradually to the highest number over a six-week period. An additional set may be added as strength and endurance increase.)

Age (in years)	Repetitions in one set
To 49	10–40
50–59	10–35
60–69	10–35
70+	10–30

ARM SWINGS

Enter the water almost at shoulder height, put your left foot in front of your right, and bend both knees so that your shoulders are beneath the water. Hold your arms straight out in front of your body, with the palms turned down.

Swing your arms down by the sides of your body and then push them behind your body, while keeping your fingers together and arms straight to increase resistance. When you have forced your arms as far behind your body as you can, rotate the arms so that your palms face forward and then move them forward again, back up to the starting position. Keep both arms completely beneath the water during the exercise.

This exercise benefits the shoulders, chest, and upper arms.

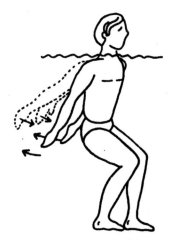

Goals for Different Age Groups (These are the number of repetitions to be performed in one set of the exercise, without interruption. Begin with the lowest number of repetitions and increase gradually to the highest number over a six-week period. An additional set may be added as strength and endurance increase.)

Age (in years)	Repetitions in one set
To 49	10–40
50–59	10–35
60–69	10–35
70+	10–30

Aqua-Aerobics for Muscle Group #2: Abdomen and Trunk

HIP SWINGS

Place your back against the pool wall, and support your body by extending your arms along the edge of the pool. Your legs should be straight out in front of your body, parallel to the bottom of the pool.

Keeping your back against the wall and your legs together, swing both legs to the left side of the wall. Contract your abdominal muscles, and swing both legs across your body toward the right side of the pool. This movement constitutes *two* repetitions (one to the left and one to the right).

This exercise strengthens the abdominal muscles and the muscles at the side of the abdomen.

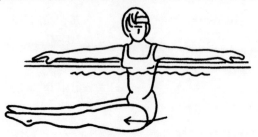

Goals for Different Age Groups (These are the number of repetitions to be performed in one set of the exercise, without interruption. Begin with the lowest number of repetitions and increase gradually to the highest number over a six-week period. An additional set may be added as strength and endurance increase.)

Age (in years)	*Repetitions in one set*
To 49	8–25
50–59	8–20
60–69	8–15
70+	5–10

WATER PEDALING

Position your back against the pool wall, and hold your body away from the edge by supporting yourself with both arms along the side of the pool. Allow your back to drift away from the wall.

Begin to pedal with your feet and legs as if you were riding a bicycle. To increase the exercise for your abdomen and waist, you can twist at the hips, back and forth from one side to the other, as you execute this movement. Keep your legs under the water in order to increase resistance. Twenty pedaling motions, ten to the right and ten to the left, constitute twenty repetitions.

This exercise strengthens the abdominal muscles.

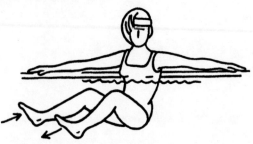

Goals for Different Age Groups (These are the number of repetitions to be performed in one set of the exercise, without interruption. Begin with

the lowest number of repetitions and increase gradually to the highest number over a six-week period. An additional set may be added as strength and endurance increase.)

Age (in years)	Repetitions in one set
To 49	20–60
50–59	20–50
60–69	20–40
70+	10–20

TWIST AND SHOUT

Bend at the knees so that your shoulders are under water, with your weight on the balls of your feet. Bend your arms at the elbows and hold them in front of you.

Move your hips back and forth, from one side to the other, and move your arms back and forth in the opposite direction from your hips. As you twist your body back and forth, keep your feet firmly planted on the bottom of the pool. One rotation counts as one repetition. You should do half of your rotation repetitions on the right side and half on the left.

This exercise strengthens most of the abdominal and lower trunk muscles.

Goals for Different Age Groups (These are the number of repetitions to be performed in one set of the exercise, without interruption. Begin with the lowest number of repetitions and increase gradually to the highest number over a six-week period. An additional set may be added as strength and endurance increase.)

Age (in years)	Repetitions in one set
To 49	20–60
50–59	20–50
60–69	20–40
70+	10–20

Aqua-Aerobics for Muscle Group #3: Legs and Lower Back

THIGH SPLITS

Position your back against the side of the pool, and extend your arms along the edge of the pool to support your body. Your legs should be held straight out in front of your body, parallel to the bottom of the pool, with your ankles flexed. Keep your abdomen tucked in, and press your lower back against the wall.

To execute the exercise, first push your legs wide apart and then pull them back together. This movement constitutes one repetition.

This exercise strengthens the muscles on the outer and inner thighs.

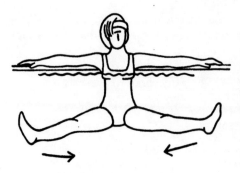

Goals for Different Age Groups (These are the number of repetitions to be performed in one set of the exercise, without interruption. Begin with the lowest number of repetitions and increase gradually to the highest number over a six-week period. An additional set may be added as strength and endurance increase.)

Age (in years)	Repetitions in one set
To 49	5–25
50–59	5–20
60–69	5–15
70+	5–10

HIGH WATER KICKS

Stand with your back against the pool wall in waist-deep water, and steady yourself using both arms on the side of the pool.

Lift your right leg straight up toward your right side, with your right ankle flexed. Swing your right leg in front of your body toward your left side. Then, swing your right leg back to the right across your body, and assume a standing position again, with both feet on the bottom of the pool. This motion constitutes one repetition. Repeat the movement in reverse with your left leg for the second repetition.

This exercise benefits the thigh and hip muscles.

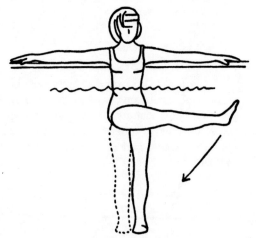

Goals for Different Age Groups (These are the number of repetitions to be performed in one set of the exercise, without interruption. Begin with the lowest number of repetitions and increase gradually to the highest number over a six-week period. An additional set may be added as strength and endurance increase.)

Age (in years)	Repetitions in one set
To 49	5–25
50–59	5–20
60–69	5–15
70+	5–10

Part Three

Entering a New
Faith-Fitness Zone

9

THE FINE-TUNING EFFECT

If you become tired of doing the same old walking, jogging, or swimming every week, there is no higher authority that says you can't vary your program every now and then. In fact, the evidence I've gathered over the years indicates that, for most people, it is essential to fine-tune exercise programs periodically to prevent them from going stale.

But if you want to add a little spice to your workout, you should bear in mind the three factors in what I call "the Fine-Tuning Effect." These include:

Factor #1: Devote at least eight weeks to reaching and maintaining a reasonable level of fitness.

Factor #2: To add variety, replace a few sessions of your regular exercise program with other activities that have similar fitness value. For example, if you're a runner, you might substitute one of your running days with distance swimming or cycling. Or if you've been using only weights for your strength training, you might switch to calisthenics for a week.

Factor #3: Feel free to take a short "vacation" from your program or to skip occasional exercise sessions.

Here's a further description of each of these factors and some explanations of how the Fine-Tuning Effect works in practice.

Fine-Tuning Factor #1: Devote at Least Eight Weeks to Your Program

I believe that every exerciser should plan on spending at least eight weeks on an exercise program before he or she thinks about making substantial changes in the routine. All that's necessary is to check what's required during the eighth or ninth week in the Beginner program that you chose in chapter seven. When you pass that point, you're ready for some fine-tuning.

In practical terms, this means that, at age forty-five, a man or woman could achieve the eight-week goal by walking three miles, four times per week, with a forty-five-minute time limit for each walking session. The same effect could be reached by jogging two miles in twenty minutes, four days per week. Or the exerciser could swim 1,300 yards three times per week, with a thirty-six minute limit for each swimming session.

Similarly, to be ready to fine-tune a strength or flexibility fitness program, you should have been on that regimen for at least eight weeks before you try any serious experimentation.

WHY IS THIS WAITING PERIOD NECESSARY?

I've found that it typically takes eight weeks to habituate or "groove" the body to a relatively high level of regular exercise and to become familiar with your body's peculiar reactions to athletic activity. After a certain period of time, your muscles and endurance capacity tend to communicate to you whether you're getting enough or too much exercise. Also, you'll be more aware of whether staying on one routine tends to bore you.

In general, putting in at least eight weeks on one regular, consistent program will lower the risk that you'll quit altogether if you find yourself becoming disappointed or distracted by trying to include variations in your routine. I've known some exercisers who started out jogging for three or four weeks and then abruptly switched to swimming, cycling, or some other sport. But they found their swimming or cycling skills weren't adequate for them to complete a full workout, and so they became discouraged and stopped working out altogether. In contrast, those who spend at least eight weeks at one activity usually find it easier to experiment with their basic program and then return to it if the attempt at a fine-tuning variation doesn't quite work out.

Furthermore, if you exercise consistently for at least eight weeks, you'll find you develop built-in physiologic responses that will encourage you to keep working out—even if trying other exercise variations becomes a little disruptive. In particular, once you get into fairly good shape, you'll discover that if you stop exercising completely for a few days, you may notice some strange symptoms. Your head may seem "fuzzy," your mental processes become unclear, and you may not sleep as well. In addition, you may experience feelings of restlessness and perhaps of being a little "down" or depressed.

These are signs of the "withdrawal" from the "positive addiction" that exercise experts have identified in well-conditioned, regular exercisers. The negative feelings and sensations that accompany a failure to exercise may be due to the absence of the body's pleasant, relaxation-producing endor-phins. These morphine-like neurotransmitters are released by the brain during exercise and may account for both the addictive effects of aerobic activity and the withdrawal symptoms that accompany its cessation.

EIGHT WEEKS AS A HEALTH INSURANCE POLICY

There's still another benefit to putting in at least eight straight weeks on your program. The longer you pursue a regular exercise routine, the stronger your position will be to bounce back from lengthy gaps that may crop up in your program.

The indications I have among my patients and other exercisers is that the better conditioned a person is, and the longer and more intensely he has followed a training regimen, the more slowly he will become deconditioned. Even if a well-conditioned person neglects his program for several weeks, he'll be able to approach his original level of fitness in less time and with less effort than those who have never been fit in the first place.

What we have here is a *delayed deconditioning* and a *quicker rebound* among those who have reached a good level of fitness, neglected their pro-gram, and then started again. Here are a couple of examples.

The Return of a Busy Executive   A fifty-four-year-old executive em-barked on a progressive program that involved walking for about two miles a day, three days a week; then jogging and walking; finally, running for four days a week. Typically, he covered two miles in twenty to twenty-two minutes, or ten to eleven minutes per mile. Three days a week, he had a simple strength/flexibility program, with stretching exercises for the back, hamstring stretches, fifty sit-ups, seven to nine chin-ups, and thirty to forty push-ups.

He stayed on this program for about four years; then downsizing and other internal turmoil at his company made it necessary for him to put in exceptionally long hours. As a result, he began to miss many of his regularly scheduled exercise sessions. For this executive, however, the change in his routine didn't reflect a decision to neglect his body. Rather, he was dem-onstrating an intensified emphasis on more important priorities in his life—namely his deep commitment to his coworkers and his occupational responsi-bilities.

But this was just a temporary adjustment. When his workload finally eased up six months later, his convictions about physical fitness helped him return to his exercise routine. Predictably, he found he couldn't run as far or as fast as in the past, or do as well with the flexibility or strength activities. But within only about three weeks, he was back up to his original jogging level and was doing as many repetitions of his calisthenics as he had achieved earlier.

The Aerobic Recovery of a New Grandmother A fifty-three-year-old woman had become an avid walker, often spending an hour or more getting to places most of her friends reached by car. She walked at least five days a week, averaging three miles at a pace of fifteen to sixteen minutes per mile. She was drawn to this activity largely because it provided her with an extended period during which she could pray for friends and family members and plan her activities for the day.

This regimen lasted for nearly ten years, but when her first grandchild was born, her exercise program took a back seat, primarily because of other beliefs, rooted in her firm religious convictions, that the needs of her family had to take precedence over her accustomed exercise-and-prayer routine. As it happened, her daughter-in-law, who had a full-time job, needed a babysitter, and the grandmother volunteered. Although she continued to walk and pray, she engaged in fewer outings over shorter distances.

These arrangements changed when the mother of the child decided to work part-time. Then, the grandmother was free to return to her regular exercise routine, but she quickly discovered that the long period of reduced exercise had resulted in considerable deconditioning. Still, after only two weeks of regular walking, her leg muscles and feet toughened up again, and in less than a month, she was back to her original level of activity.

There appear to be at least three reasons for the positive experiences of this executive and grandmother:

- Both had deep convictions about the importance of fitness.
- Neither stopped exercising completely. Improving fitness is always easier and more rapid than starting a program from a state of complete inactivity.
- Those who have been in good shape at some relatively recent point in the past seem to harbor a confident expectation about returning to the former fitness level.

There's obviously a limit to this last concept. A person who was athletic as a teenager but then becomes sedentary for twenty years will lose all his conditioning and will have to start at the very beginning with any sort of exercise program. But a trained exerciser who cuts back for a few weeks or months should find that regaining good shape can be accomplished in a relatively short period of time.

Of course, I don't cite these illustrations to suggest that you should reduce or give up your program for several months as these people did. But such examples *do* demonstrate that a previously well-conditioned body can be returned to something near its original condition in a relatively short period of time—provided the layoff hasn't been excessively long.

So there are many benefits to sticking with your exercise program for at least eight weeks. If you do fulfill this commitment, you'll find that you can vary your program in ways that will make the regimen considerably more interesting and effective.

Fine-Tuning Factor #2: Begin to Substitute Other Athletic Activities in Your Regular Exercise Program

Once you've reached a reasonable level of aerobic and strength-flexibility fitness, and maintained it for at least eight weeks, you're ready to try adding a little variation to your program. I know that those who are disciplined, nose-to-the-grindstone exercisers may become a little nervous here. Sometimes, I'll hear questions like these:

- "If I change my program—or worse, start doing easier exercises—won't I become lax and lose my fitness?"
- "I want to get in *better* shape, not back off on my program. How will this idea help me?"
- "I've worked hard to reach this level of conditioning, and I'm satisfied with what I've achieved. Why should I fool around with a good thing?"

These are all good questions, and certainly, it's not necessary to change your program if you really don't want to. But I've discovered that many well-conditioned individuals who have been on the same regimen for several months or years are eager to try something new. In short, they need a little extra spice in their exercise life.

If you're in this category, the Fine-Tuning Effect may be just the thing for you. And the first move you should consider making is inserting a new activity into your program, even if it seems initially to be less demanding than your original sport. The chances are, if you make your substitutions wisely, you'll end up more motivated than ever, with a much stronger program than you had before the fine-tuning began. That's what happened with one of my patients when he moved from New York City to Florida.

GIL'S TRIPLE THREAT

Gil, a self-employed businessman in his early fifties, had jogged for years on the streets of Manhattan and had developed a level of endurance

A Lesson in How Not to Vary Your Exercise—By C. S. Lewis

The Cambridge don and popular Christian philosopher, C. S. Lewis, was a great walker, and he enjoyed sharing his walks with others who could carry on a stimulating conversation. But on one occasion, he made the mistake of varying one of his outings by taking along a less than compatible companion. Here are some excerpts from a letter he wrote to his brother on March 20, 1932:

> You asked Mrs. Moore in a recent letter about this Crashaw man. . . . I had to go for a walk with him. . . . It seemed good to him to take a bus to the station and start our walk along a sort of scrubby path between a factory and a greasy strip of water. . . . He is a ladylike little man of about fifty, and is to a T that "sensible, well-informed man" with whom Lamb dreaded to be left alone. . . . I blundered at once by referring to the water as a canal. "Oh, could it be that I didn't know it was the Thames? Perhaps I was not a walker?" . . .
>
> A conversation on weather followed, and seemed to offer an escape from unmitigated fact. The escape however was quite illusory and my claim to be rather fond of all sorts of weather was received with the stunning information that psychologists detected the same trait in children and lunatics. Anxious to turn my attention from this unpleasing fact, he begged my opinion of various changes which had recently been made in the river; indeed every single lock, bridge, and style has apparently been radically altered in the last few months. As I had never seen any of the places before ("But I thought you said you were a walker . . ?") this bowled me middle stump again. . . .
>
> But I must stop my account of this deplorable walk somewhere. It was the same all through—sheer information. Time after time I attempted to get away from the torrent of isolated, particular facts; but anything tending to opinion, a discussion, to fancy, to ideas, even to putting some of his infernal facts together and making something out of them—anything of that sort was received in blank silence.
>
> —from W.H. Lewis, ed., *Letters of C.S. Lewis*
> (New York: Harcourt Brace Jovanovich, 1966), pp. 150–151.

Lessons from Lewis on exercising with a companion:

- One of the best motivators for sticking with an exercise program is to find a "soulmate" who can make you look forward to each outing.
- One of the biggest deterrents to an exercise program is to dread having to meet a companion who is "out of sync" with you. I expect that if Lewis had been forced to face the prospect of walking with this particular man every day, he would have given up walking altogether and perhaps turned to a treadmill instead!

that enabled him to score consistently in the top, "superior" category on our treadmill stress tests at the Cooper Clinic. But during the past four years, partly through boredom and partly from the increasing demands of his work, he cut his weekly running mileage back from about twelve miles to six per week. He did play doubles tennis two or three times a month and singles squash about three times a month, and he consistently walked a total of two miles daily between his apartment and his office. But this combination of relatively light exercises wasn't enough to keep up his superior level of endurance.

According to our stress test records, Gil dropped down to the "excellent" category for two straight checkups—which was still commendable, but not up to the standards he had set for himself. Also, I was concerned that this downward trend in his conditioning might continue.

Another problem that Gil faced was spiritual. When he had first started running, he had used his outings of at least two to three miles per day, four to five days a week, to extend his private prayer time. Now, the shorter periods he was spending in endurance activity meant he had less time for these devotions.

Gil's exercise and devotional life changed unexpectedly for the better when he decided to move his business operation to Florida. Because he lived close to the Atlantic Ocean, he was able to continue his jogging program on the beach, and he found the beautiful setting made him want to run for longer distances of two to three miles. Just the change of scene had rejuvenated his endurance efforts. As an added benefit, the longer outings and the closeness to nature inspired him to resume his prayer time during exercise.

To enhance the flavor of his endurance program, Gil also started including bicycling and distance swimming in his workouts. He worked up to a level of skill in both these new endurance sports that enabled him to get cardiovascular benefits that were similar to what he achieved with running. On a given day he might not feel like running, but cycling might seem appealing. Or he might go for a run and then cap it off with a quarter-mile to half-mile swim to cool off. Or on days when he was really feeling ambitious, he would do all three sports, which he called his "triple threat" against boredom.

I realize that you may not be able to move to another part of the country to find more opportunities for interesting variations on your exercise routine. But I would encourage you to think more creatively about how to structure your fitness program. Undoubtedly, there are two or three possibilities that are literally begging for your response, so why wait to take advantage of them?

I vary my own approach by running a few days each week on the Cooper Aerobics Center track, which passes right in front of my office. But on those days I don't run, I'll go out for a fast walk after work with my wife, Millie, or with our little dog, whom I carry in my arms for the two miles I cover on the streets around our home. On vacations and holidays, I'll substitute hiking, mountain climbing, or mountain biking.

The challenge is to find at least two or three endurance and strength activities which are convenient to do where you live or work, and which you can make a commitment to pursue on a regular basis. Once you develop several parallel exercise possibilities, boredom will become a thing of the past.

Fine-Tuning Factor #3: If You're Feeling Stale or Fatigued, Take a Short Vacation from Exercise, or Skip an Occasional Workout

Yona is a forty-seven-year-old woman who was a committed marathon runner. She wasn't a champion competitor, but she ran in several marathons each year and often covered ten to eighteen miles per day in training.

Both she and I expected her to perform exceptionally well on the treadmill stress test when she came in for a checkup. To score in the superior category for her age group, she would have had to walk twenty minutes on the test, and I thought she would easily better that. In fact, I predicted she had a good chance to top twenty-six or twenty-seven minutes.

I was considerably off the mark. She actually came in slightly *under* twenty minutes, a performance that placed her in the excellent category for women her age. That was certainly a top-level result, but far below what I would have expected for a woman so highly conditioned.

What went wrong? I immediately decided that she was overloading her muscles by working out so strenuously. She just didn't seem to be getting enough rest, and so she was unable to do her best. As an antidote, I suggested that she actually lay off her exercise routine for a week and then come in for another stress test. She took my advice, and the next week, she walked on the treadmill for more than twenty-five minutes, which was a new personal record.

The lesson we should learn from this woman's experience is that it's perfectly all right to take some time off from a vigorous exercise program, especially if you're feeling chronic fatigue or listlessness. It may just be that you're working out too hard and you need to pull back to allow your body time to recover. In other words, you are no longer training; you are *straining.* Also, it's essential to do a personal evaluation of yourself every so often to be sure that you're keeping your exercise routine in perspective with the rest of your life.

One of the most overlooked problems of serious older amateur athletes is that they typically have other responsibilities and interests involving their work or families. In trying to live up to all these commitments *and* to their exercise goals, they run out of time. Too often, their sleep is shortchanged. Or they may settle for hurried or poorly planned meals and fail to focus on good nutrition. Without enough sleep or a proper diet, fatigue or a feeling of being run down is inevitable.

The best answer in such a situation is for the athlete to take a short vacation from exercise. Usually, I recommend that the layoff be limited to one week, and in many cases, it only takes three or four days for high energy levels to return.

Second, after the vacation has been completed, I may suggest that the athlete exercise less intensely. A person like Yona, for example, would probably *gain* in conditioning and performance if she cut her long daily runs in half—say, down to about five to eight miles—with an occasional longer distance when she's in training for a specific race. It often takes some experimentation to find out if cutting back on the intensity or frequency of a workout will improve performance.

Studies among a variety of athletes of every age, including intercollegiate swimmers as well as middle-age runners, have shown that reducing exercise can enhance competitive times. One of the main reasons for this phenomenon is that working out too much can deplete the all-important stores of glycogen or sugar in the body. This development deprives the muscles of the energy resources they need to sustain a peak level of performance.

In contrast, cutting back on the training routine can give the body a chance to build up its glycogen stores. The end results are often greater feelings of physical comfort and improvements in performance. Did you ever notice how much easier you can run on Monday, after laying off on the weekend? That's because your body is more rested and your energy reservoirs have been replenished.

THE ONE-OUT-OF-SIX RULE

Finally, I recommend that the over-forty athlete occasionally skip an entire exercise session just to be sure that the body is fully rested and fatigue is held at bay. A helpful rule that some older athletes follow is what I call the "one-out-of-six rule." The idea is to follow your regular training routine for six straight sessions, and after that, skip a session. After you skip the next workout, begin counting again, and when you reach six, skip another workout.

If you prefer *not* to skip a session immediately after you've completed six consecutive workouts, you certainly don't have to! Many people, including myself, go through periods when they really *want* to continue exercising regularly or even daily. You may be working out at a level that doesn't cause fatigue, and in fact, the activity may be helping you to feel great. But if you exercise daily, you should alternate the intensity of activity, such as by performing a hard workout one day and a lighter workout the next.

One final word for recreational or noncompetitive athletes: I advise that those in this category not exercise six or seven days per week. The risk of injury and excessive fatigue is too great for the rewards received. Four or five days is completely adequate.

There are many ways to fine-tune an exercise program, and the older a person becomes, the more essential it is to allow for sessions with less intensity or simply to take a short vacation from the routine. I realize, of course, that varying the rigor of a routine may be a very difficult balancing act for some people. The danger is that the fine-tuner may gradually begin to cut back more and more on his program until he eventually loses his top level of conditioning.

But most of the time, the benefits will far outweigh this risk for those who have established a firm exercise base and who regularly test their levels of fitness to be sure they are not slipping. As those of us who have been at this for years know, the sense of well-being that accompanies regular, challenging physical conditioning is usually enough in itself to provide insurance against the cardinal sin of falling forever from a state of high fitness.

10

THE UNLIMITED
PERFORMANCE PRINCIPLE

We should *never* try to place a ceiling on the body's potential because of age. I believe that we can *all* push back our physical limits—just as Abraham did, when, even though he was well past one hundred, he made the arduous journey to Egypt and negotiated with the pharaoh.

My convictions about your possibilities—which is summed up in what I've called the Unlimited Performance Principle—applies across the board to the thirty-plus population. The main idea is never to sell yourself short. Instead, so long as you gain medical clearance before attempting new heights of achievement, you can often do more than what any "expert" says you can.

Let me emphasize, though, that in stating this principle, I'm *not* just talking about those older athletes who are capable of playing or performing at a world-class level. Sometimes athletic achievement must be measured not by how well you do in a particular event, but just by *whether or not you can finish what you start!*

How far can you expect to go in increasing your physical performance after you pass age thirty or forty?

We've already seen in chapter 4 how you can lower your Real Age by recapturing endurance levels and other athletic capacities that you enjoyed as a youth. We've explored in chapter 9 how the Fine-Tuning Effect can not only make exercise more enjoyable and relaxing but may also improve competitive performance.

To complete our discussion about what's possible as you grow older, let's consider how several representative athletes have tested the outer limits of athletic performance in older age groups.

Extending the Championship Season

In a number of cases, former athletic greats have succeeded at maintaining high performance well past age forty. Here are a few cases that have piqued my interest:

- Frank Havens at age twenty-seven was an Olympic gold medal winner in the 10,000-meter canoe race. At age sixty-two, he was still competing and could beat his gold medal time by one minute!
- Henry Marsh, a four-time Olympian and American record holder for the 3,000-meter steeplechase, didn't run his first sub-four-minute mile until he was thirty-two years of age.
- David Costill, captain of the Ohio University men's swim team in 1957–58, turned in top times of 02:23 for the 200-yard individual medley and 02:07 for the 200-yard freestyle. After age forty-six, he had actually improved: He did the medley in 02:16 and the freestyle in 01:59. Even by age fifty-three, he was faster in every swimming event in which he had competed at age twenty.
- Al Oerter was the four-time Olympic discus gold medalist in the 1956, 1960, 1964, and 1968 games.

Now in his late fifties, Oerter last won the Olympics when he was thirty-two. But he's continued to stay in shape and holds several masters records in the discus. In fact, up until his late forties, Oerter's masters records were comparable to, and in some instances greater than, his Olympic throws!

"The effect of age in weight throwing appears to be quite minimal," Oerter said at age fifty-two in a 1988 symposium conducted by the *NSCA Journal.* "I can train as long (around two hours), as often (seven days per week), and with as much intensity as ever. My goals have lowered somewhat, and I no longer have the Olympics in mind each time I train. I have replaced this with world masters championships and as much open (all ages) competition as I find comfortable."

Oerter has also followed his own version of the Fine-Tuning Effect by making age-related changes in his routine: "When I was a teenager, through my twenties, I lifted heavily every other day. Since that time, I have rested for two days between heavy sessions. One of those days is utilized for light supportive exercise."

The solid base of athletic workouts has also given him the freedom to skip workouts or take a vacation from his activities without ill effect. "I have thrown every other day for most of my athletic career. If I don't feel like lifting or throwing, I just take time off. This can be two to three days or, in one instance, eight years. If it's not there, I just don't believe in forcing it."

I wouldn't recommend an eight-year layoff for most older athletes! But the principle of taking a *limited* amount of time off from a regular routine is quite sound.

Another interesting and, I believe, healthy change that takes place in many of these world-class athletes is that even though winning is still important, it's not everything. They have already accomplished a great deal, and they don't have to prove anything to themselves or to others. As a result, they begin to get more of a kick out of the competition *and* the training.

Al Oerter finds that among older world-class athletes, there is the "same goal setting, willingness to put in the required work, the [wonderful] feeling of competing with folks of a similar mind, testing oneself."

Oerter provides a sound philosophy of athletic competition for those of us who are well past college age when he gives this advice:

> When you're tired, stop. When you don't feel like it, don't. When you're injured, rest. When "things" invade training time, take care of them first. Stop to feel the sun [and] wind. The rest of the time, hit it! (From "Roundtable: Training the older athlete, Part II—Practical considerations," *NSCA Journal*, Vol. 10, Number 6, 1988, pp. 10–14.)

THE THREE MAIN FACTORS THAT CAUSE DECLINE

So what are we to conclude from these observations? I'd sum things up this way:

- In part, the decline in performance over time stems from a diminishing intensity of motivation. Winning is just not that important any more!
- In part, the decline may come from a tendency to cut back on the intensity of workouts, beyond the top level of performance that can be sustained by the Fine-Tuning Effect.
- In part, the decline in performance among older top athletes is an inevitable function of age.

Even highly committed competitive runners experience about a 5 to 10 percent loss in their times up to age forty. Older swimmers seem to lose even more, but in part, this loss can be traced to the fact that they don't have the time to put in the long hours in the pool and weight room.

For example, Roger Cundall, a former swimmer at the University of Southern California, found that, at age forty-four, his times in the 100-yard breaststroke were ten seconds slower than his times in college. On the other hand, in the first stages of his comeback at age forty-two, former Olympic gold medalist Mark Spitz was able to come within a couple of seconds of world-class time in the short freestyle distances.

Age, then, will certainly cut into athletic performance. But maintaining desire and training intensity can reduce the rate of the decline well into older age.

THE MOTIVATION FACTOR AFTER FORTY

How can you keep your motivation and training intensity at a high level as you grow older? I'd suggest several guidelines that have worked for me and other older athletes I know:

Guideline #1: Recognize that your competitive drive will probably diminish—and accept it! Most people become mellower as they age; they may like to win, but a victory in a sports event just isn't the most important thing in their lives any more. It's important to accept this development and not feel guilty or try to manufacture enthusiasm that just isn't there. This sort of anxiety-producing behavior will produce unnecessary stress and work against the psychological benefits of a fitness program.

Guideline #2: Set realistic fitness goals that you'd like to maintain for the rest of your life. You can't be an Olympic athlete when you're eighty or ninety, but you *can* achieve and stay at a superior level of aerobic and strength/flexibility fitness. Decide what that level is and strive toward it, but don't worry if you fall a little short of your expectations. Just the fact that you're remaining quite active will reduce your overall risk of disease and early death.

It's also possible that you'll have to adjust your fitness goals downward somewhat as you move through your seventies, eighties, or nineties, just because of the natural decline in performance that accompanies aging. But then again, maybe you won't! Because so much is still unknown about the performance potential of older people, I'm inclined to keep expectations high rather than low—so long as high physical achievement is something you really want. The main thing that we do know is that no arbitrary limits should be placed on the physical potential of those over forty.

Guideline #3: Identify the level of exercise intensity and frequency required for you to maintain your fitness goals. This is probably the most crucial step in keeping up a reasonably high degree of fitness in your later years. Yet to take this step, you must have the facts. You need to know how far and fast you have to run, swim, or cycle—and how many repetitions of certain strength and flexibility exercises you must do—to stay at your target level of fitness.

If you're committed to competitive athletics or just want to reach your highest physical potential, a simple way to find whether your exercise intensity and frequency are working is to test your outer physical limits every six months or so. If your favorite event is the mile, see how fast you can run it. Or suppose you compete in the 100-yard freestyle: Every few months try a test race to check how fast you can cover that distance. If you find you're slipping in your test performance, increase your training intensity, or frequency, or both. Then, if you're back up to your target level at the next testing period, you'll know you're on the right track.

Caution: If you're working out at a high level of intensity, be sure to monitor your level of fatigue or muscle soreness, and cut back on your exercise as much as possible to minimize these discomforts. Also, to prevent the effects of harmful "free radicals" (unstable oxygen molecules produced by excessive exercise), take antioxidant supplements according to the recommendations in chapter 4 of my book *Antioxidant Revolution* (Thomas Nelson, 1994).

Guideline #4: If your interest or motivation declines with one fitness activity, switch to another.

A Judicial Solution. Here's a case in point: John, a prominent judge in one of our larger cities, discovered competitive running when he was in his forties. He competed in dozens of races, including several marathons. But by the time he reached his late fifties, he was "burned out on roadwork," to use his term.

John had suffered several injuries from the pounding that his body had taken from his intense training and the demands of racing. The discomfort had detracted from the pleasure he had originally derived from running. Just as important, he was looking for new fields to conquer, new physical challenges. So he switched to rowing.

John still jogs a couple of days a week, but he goes for much shorter distances and at a slower pace than when he was training for competitive distance running. He spends at least three days a week on a river near his home working out in a racing scull. And he exercises on a stationary rowing machine that he has set up in his home.

Treadmill tests show that John has maintained his superior aerobic capacity, even though he has switched sports. He has also increased his strength and flexibility as a result of the upper-body demands of the rowing.

Perhaps most important of all, John's motivation to maintain a rigorous physical fitness program has returned in full force. He's still learning the techniques of his new skill, and it seems likely that he'll be at this sport for years to come. If his interest in rowing begins to wane, I know John has learned an important lesson: He will be off on still *another* new athletic tangent which will continue to keep him in great shape as he ages.

Many of my older athletic patients have had down times comparable to John's, and they have seen their enthusiasm return when they move from running to cycling or triathalons. The experience of these individuals confirms the importance of still another dimension of the Fine-Tuning Effect: By making adjustments in your program as you age—and especially by following new athletic interests—you'll add excitement to your fitness activities and enhance your desire to keep performing at a high level.

But even after an older athlete has made these adjustments, the question still remains: What are my limits? As I've indicated, each person's ultimate capacity will be different. But here are some ideas about how far it's possible to go as you age.

A Mountaintop Experience

Francesco Petrarca, commonly known today as Petrarch, was a fourteenth-century European scholar and philosopher and a decisive figure in ushering in the age of the Renaissance. Born in southern France of Italian parents, he was deeply religious, even in his younger years, and in his mid-twenties he underwent a profound spiritual experience during an arduous climb with his brother of Mount Ventoux in southern France. He described this experience in a letter written on April 26, 1336, to a revered teacher. Here are some words from his account:

Today I ascended the highest mountain in this region, which, not without cause, they call the Windy Peak. Nothing but the desire to see its conspicuous height was the reason to make this expedition. . . .

The day was long, the air was mild; this and vigorous minds, strong and supple bodies, and all the other conditions assisted us on our way. . . . We . . . began to climb with merry alacrity. However, as almost always happens, the daring attempt was soon followed by quick fatigue.

Not far from our start we stopped at a rock. From there we went on again, proceeding at a slower pace, to be sure. I in particular made my way up with considerably more modest steps. My brother endeavored to reach the summit by the very ridge of the mountain on a short cut; I, being so much more of a weakling, was bending down toward the valley. When he called me back and showed me the better way, I answered that I hoped to find an easier access on the other side. . . . With such an excuse I tried to palliate my laziness, and, when the others had already reached the higher zones, I was still wandering through the valleys, where no more comfortable access was revealed, while the way became longer and longer and the vain fatigue grew heavier and heavier.

Two more times, Petrarca tried to find an easier route to the top, and two more times he failed—to his brother's great amusement. Finally, the young philosopher drew a connection between his physical efforts and his spiritual life:

I leaped in my winged thoughts from things corporeal to what is incorporeal and addressed myself in words like these:

"What you have so often experienced today while climbing this mountain happens to you, you must know, and to many others who are making their way toward the blessed life. This is not easily understood by us men, because the motions of the body lie open, while those of the mind are invisible and hidden. The life we call blessed is located on a high peak. 'A narrow way,' they say, leads up to it. Many hilltops intervene, and we must proceed 'from virtue to virtue' with exalted steps. On the highest summit is set the end of all, the goal toward which our pilgrimage is directed. . . . What is it then that keeps you back? Evidently nothing but the smoother way that leads through the meanest earthly pleasures and looks easier at first sight. However, having strayed far in error, you must either ascend to the summit of the blessed life under the heavy burden of hard striving . . . or lie prostrate in your slothfulness in the valleys. . . ."

You cannot imagine how much comfort this thought brought my mind and body for what lay still ahead of me. Would that I might achieve with my mind the journey for which I am longing day and night, as I achieved with the feet . . . my journey today, after overcoming all obstacles. . . .

There is a summit, higher than all the others. . . . On its top is a small level stretch. There at last we rested from our fatigue.

—from Francesco Petrarca, "The Ascent of Mont Ventoux," in *The Renaissance Philosophy of Many,* ed. by Ernst Cassirer, et al. (Chicago: The University of Chicago Press, 1948, 1961), pp. 36–46.

Lessons from Petrarca:

- The way to physical achievement—including good health and fitness—requires work and discipline. You have to map out a plan and stick to it if you want to reach the "summit" of good condition and energetic living.
- The way to the spiritual summit—that is, the profound inner development and maturity that may arise upon the foundation of a serious, heartfelt spiritual commitment—also requires consistency and discipline.
- When you embark on your daily exercise program, don't be limited by the huffing and puffing of the physical effort. Look beyond the responses of your body and try to discern insights that can nurture your spirit.

THE LIMITS OF PERFORMANCE

In exploring more precisely what the physical limits of aging humans may be, I like to think in terms of three basic questions: How far? How fast, high, or long? How old?

How far? There are apparently no limits as to distance or endurance for over-forty athletes. The so-called "ultramarathoners" are proof of this fact.

What's an ultramarathon? Some argue that it's a continuous footrace longer than a marathon. But I go along with the ultramarathon scribe and athlete John L. Parker, who presents a looser definition: He applies the term to any race or event that is longer than the 26-mile 385-yard marathon, even though the distance may be covered in stages or over a period of days, with rest periods in between.

A few illustrations demonstrate how well older people perform at these longer, sometimes incredible, distances:

Helen Klein, the Sixty-Eight-Year-Old Grandmother. Helen began serious running at age fifty-five and during her sixties has graduated to distances of fifty to one hundred-plus miles. Her goal every time she enters an event is just to finish, she says, and she's done an excellent job of that.

For example, she ran the Jed Smith fifty-miler in Sacramento in nine hours and one minute in 1984. She ran the Vermont 100-miler in 24:59:00 in 1989, at the age of sixty-six. And she did the Western States 100 in 29:25:00 in 1989.

Imagine! A woman in her late sixties moving continuously on her feet for more than a full day! She told *Ultrarunning* magazine (Nov. 1990) that a couple of motivational factors make these huge distances fun for her:

> Finishing races give you such a wonderful sense of accomplishment and makes you feel good about yourself. But the greatest reason is that Norman [her husband, a leading ultra-race director] is so involved because we've always done everything together (p. 36).

Again, we're reminded of how important motivation is for every athlete. Working out with a friend or family member—or just knowing that you're supported in your efforts—can make all the difference in sticking with a fitness program.

An interesting side note involving Klein: During the course of her ultramarathon efforts, she has discovered the significance of upper-body strength training. One major 100-mile event, the Old Dominion, involved a long upward climb. The first time she tried this ascent, she says:

> I had to stop a few times to breathe, and I wrongfully assumed it was my lungs. Actually, as the race medical director pointed out to me, the problem was the muscles that support my shoulders. I didn't have upper body strength. I needed to work on those muscles to support me so that I had better posture going up (p. 35).

So she joined a health club and starting doing upper body and abdominal exercises. The next time she tried the Old Dominion, she reported, "Climbing is still difficult, but now I can ascend two miles without resting."

Otto Appenzeller, the Ultra-Running Physician. Appenzeller, at sixty years of age, was running seventy to ninety miles per week in his training. He founded the 28½-mile Sandia Wilderness Crossing Research Run in New Mexico and has used it to investigate the effects of aerobic training on the human nervous system.

He was in his early fifties when he ran his first ultramarathon, a 52-mile event from London to Brighton in Great Britain. Like Helen Klein, he has competed in the Western States 100-mile race, with a top time for this distance of 25:20:00.

The 350-mile Trans-Indiana Run. This one-time event, run in 1985, involved ten over-forty athletes, including the oldest, sixty-four-year-old Dr. Howard Henry, and my friend Hal Higdon, who was in his mid-fifties at the time.

The objective was to cover the length of Indiana in ten days on foot. Higdon recorded his experiences in John L. Parker, Jr.'s *And Then the Vulture*

Eats You—Ultramarathons: Journeys of Discovery. The experience was excruciating physically but also a testimony to how much the older body can endure.

The ten participants alternated walking and running and made up their own schedules as to when they would stop to eat or sleep for a few hours. The way stations included naps in farmhouses; handouts and waterhoses from sympathetic suburban spectators; and snacks at local diners. Seven managed to finished in the alloted ten days, and only three dropped out. Higdon and Henry were among the seven "first-place finishers."

Despite the accomplishment, there was a physical price to pay. Several of the runners began to show serious signs of wear and tear by the eighth day. Higdon developed a swollen ankle that plagued him through the end, but the injury didn't keep him from finishing the last twenty-six miles (about a marathon's distance) in four hours. A medical exam immediately after the race revealed that he had incurred a stress fracture of his right tibia (the large inner bone of the leg, running from the knee to the ankle).

The doctor ordered no running for the next four weeks, but Higdon wasn't concerned: "I take the news calmly," he said, "since I figure I've done enough running in the last ten days to last me at least that long. I'll swim, cycle, lift weights and survive to run again."

Higdon, who has participated in more than one hundred marathons, pursues a rigorous routine: He runs seven miles, six to seven times per week, and in the winter, he's an avid cross-country skier. When he came into the Cooper Clinic for testing at age fifty-five, he achieved a superior performance on the treadmill for men of any age by walking for thirty minutes and sixteen seconds. In other words, his performance placed him in the top one percent of more than 120,000 treadmill runs.

How fast, high, or long? Most older, competitive runners agree that, as we age, speed falls off more than endurance. Speed results from a combination of stride length, frequency, and efficiency, but it appears that stride length may be tougher to maintain than stride frequency or efficiency. Exercises designed to stretch the quadriceps (the muscle group on the front of the leg, between the knee and the groin) may counteract the loss in range of motion. If such exercises prove effective, running speed, high jump, and long jump performances may improve.

Here's an indication of where the best older athletes recently stood according to masters records for some older age groups—and how they measured up to existing world records:

For men:
- The 100-meter dash record for forty-year-old men was 10.6 sec. (The world record was 9.85 sec.)

- The mile run record for men over forty was 03:58.05. (The world record was 03:44.39.)
- The high jump record for forty-year-old men was 6 ft. 9 in. (The world record was 8 ft. ½ in.)
- The long jump record for forty-year-old men was 24 ft. 9 in. (The world record was 29 ft. 4½ in.)
- The sixteen-pound shot put record for forty-year-old men was 70 ft. 3 in. (The world record was 75 ft. 10¼ in.)
- The javelin throw record for forty-two-year-old men was 259 ft. 1 in. (The world record was 313 ft. 10 in.)

For women:
- The 100-meter dash record for forty-one-year-old women was 12 sec. (The world record was 10.49 sec.)
- The mile run record for forty-year-old women was 04:54.69. (The world record was 04:15.61.)
- The high jump record for forty-two-year-old women was 5 ft. 5¾ in. (The world record was 6 ft. 10¼ in.)
- The long jump record for forty-year-old women was 20 ft. 1¼ in. (The world record was 24 ft. 8¼ in.)
- The eight-pound shot put record for forty-one-year-old women was 62 ft. 10½ in. (The world record was 74 ft. 3 in.)
- The javelin throw record (600 grams) for forty-year-old women was 170 ft. 1 in. (The world record was 262 ft. 5 in.)

I expect that, as today's younger athletes age and begin to compete in masters competitions, the records for older athletes will improve significantly. Their advanced training methods and expectations of world-class performances at older ages will undoubtedly carry them to new thresholds of physical accomplishment.

But an even more intriguing issue is this: Until what age can a person expect to maintain top-level athletic performance? Or to put it another way, how old is too old for this type of demanding competition?

How old? The octogenarian distance runner Johnny Kelley is one of the best arguments I know to enable us to respond, "You're *never* too old!"

Johnny, who is also one of my patients, has been featured on the front page of *The Wall Street Journal, USA Today,* and numerous other publications as "the marathon man." Now in his late eighties, he ran in the Boston Marathon sixty-one times and won the race twice. He also competed in the 1936 and 1948 Olympics. His best marathon time was 02:30:00, which he clocked in 1943, as the second-place finisher in the Boston event. But even in 1990, at age eighty-two, he finished the race in 05:05:00.

His training regimen has remained fairly constant, though the intensity has decreased. He runs an hour and fifteen minutes a day, six days per week, without focusing on trying to cover any definite distance or moving at any particular speed. He recently reported that even though he runs for as long a period during his workouts as he did in 1983, he doesn't run as fast.

Johnny first came in for an examination at our Clinic in 1983, and he's had eight complete exams with us. The first time, when he was in his mid-seventies, his treadmill time was twenty-four minutes; his resting heart rate was 52; his maximum heart rate during exercise was 159 beats per minute; and his weight was 135 pounds.

During his 1990 checkup, his treadmill time had dropped to sixteen minutes (still a great time for an eighty-three-year-old); his resting heart rate was 51 (an improvement!); his maximum heart rate was 149; and he weighed 134¾ pounds.

Obviously, Johnny Kelley is in great shape for a man in his eighties. But I still find myself asking, what was the cause for the decline in his aerobic performance, and can anything be done to delay that decline?

My tentative answer comes in several parts:

1. Johnny might work at increasing his muscle mass. Although Johnny's weight has remained almost exactly the same, the composition of that weight had changed over the last eight to nine years. Specifically, his percent of body fat was 14.85 percent in 1983, and it rose to 17.78 percent in 1990. What this means is that the amount of muscle tissue in his body went down and the amount of fat went up—a natural process as we age, but one which can be retarded through strength training.

You might think that it's a little silly to encourage an octogenarian who is in such superior shape to get in even better shape. But I take my cue from Johnny and what he seems to want to continue to achieve. As is already evident from our previous discussions of strength training, it's possible even for those in their nineties to experience a significant increase in muscle mass with weight training. With upper-body work, Johnny might decrease his percent of body fat *and* improve his running performance (as Helen Klein, the ultra-marathoner, did). My point is, why settle for less than your maximum capacity and performance if you have a choice?

2. Johnny might increase his running intensity slightly. He might try running a little faster, even if only for one mile of his workout. Or he might add an extra ten or fifteen minutes to his program. He's apparently backed off during the past eight years, but that may be more his choice than the demands of age. By intensifying his running program a little more, he might recover much of the aerobic capacity that he's lost.

3. Johnny might embark on a somewhat different athletic adventure to "juice up" his motivation. Now, this may seem *really* presumptuous, for me to suggest that a man who has entered sixty-one Boston Marathons needs motivation. But there is some reason that his times have declined, and that reason may be his own desire and hunger, rather than the aging process. The only way to find out is to experiment.

In particular, I wonder about the decline in his maximum heart rate and his treadmill times. It may be that these changes are entirely due to the aging process. But it may also be that part or most of the decline resulted from the fact that he's a little tired of doing treadmill tests and decided to quit before he reached exhaustion.

What changes could Johnny make? I'm *not* saying that he should give up his long-distance work or his marathon events. Rather, he might consider *adding* other events to his main interest. For example, he might try including competition at shorter distances in some of the masters events. Or his upper-body strength work might lead to another activity, such as a racquet sport.

None of this is theoretical, by the way. The masters records show dramatic strength and speed performances for those who are considerably older than Johnny Kelley. Here is a sampling from some recent masters records reports:

- The 100-meter record for ninety-year-old men was 19.9 seconds—and men up to ninety-five are still competing!
- The one-mile record for ninety-one-year-old men was 12:45.6, a mark held by Herb Kirk of Michigan, who also held the 100-yard dash record for ninety-year-olds!
- The eight-pound shot put record for ninety-five-year-old men was held by Tom Lane of California at 15 ft. 1¼ in.
- The long jump record for ninety-five-year-old men was 5 ft. 10 in., an achievement by Collister Wheeler of Oregon, who also held the high jump mark for ninety-two-year-olds of 2 ft. 9½ in.

And that was not all for Wheeler: He held the 600-gram javelin record for ninety-six-year-old men at 39 ft. Among other things, his versatile achievements showed that both lower-body and upper-body power are well within the reach of the oldest athletes.

Women also compete in the masters competitions well up into their eighties and turn in outstanding performances—such as an 8 ft. 3 in. record for the 6-pound shot put set by eighty-six-year-old Mary Ames of California. The outer physical limits for any woman or any age depend only on the inner potential given to her by God.

But if you are a sedentary, out-of-shape female, don't be intimidated or discouraged by accounts of great athletic prowess. Also, don't think you have to take these elite sportswomen as your models. It's certainly not necessary to become a masters competitor to get the most out of exercise. In fact, even if you are a total couch potato—as I was when I started with my own adult fitness program—your possibilities for enhanced health and fitness are most likely far beyond anything you can now imagine. A relatively slow, gradual, and painless program, such as those described in chapters 5 through 8, can produce such dramatic results that you'll soon be on your way to becoming your own special version of "superwoman." But as you'll see, even superwomen have to become aware of special gender-specific considerations and potential dangers as they pursue a personal fitness regimen.

11

THE SECRETS OF BECOMING
A SUPERWOMAN

The proven benefits of exercise and good nutrition have prompted more and more women in their thirties and beyond to get involved in regular fitness programs. Like men, they have been convinced by the promises of physical conditioning for general health, such as an increase in energy levels and a decrease in risk factors for diseases that can debilitate or cut life short.

There's nothing new about the presence of vibrant, vigorous women, of course. Both the Old and New Testaments abound with accounts of dynamic, action-oriented women. For example, remember Deborah, the judge; Jael, the assassin of Sisera the Canaanite; Ruth, who traveled great distances with her mother-in-law Naomi and worked long, arduous hours in the fields of her husband-to-be, Boaz; Joanna, who accompanied and helped support Jesus on his journeys with his disciples; and the Macedonian textile entrepreneur Lydia, who cared for Paul and his entourage.

Where did these women find their great energy? First, their power came from within, from God. Also, they seemed to be constantly on the go, and as we know, regular exercise increases the body's ability to perform.

Recent scientific evidence has added a number of important special considerations that active women should keep in mind as they design a personal fitness program. These considerations, which will be discussed in greater detail later in this chapter, include the following recommendations:

- Focus even more than men on total body conditioning, including strength work, to prevent loss of muscle mass and functioning. (See Special Consideration #1 described later in this chapter.)
- Limit running to no more than fifteen miles per week if you're a recreational exerciser, or thirty miles per week if you're a competitive female athlete. (See Special Consideration #2.)

- Keep your body fat between 12 and 22 percent of your total body weight. (See Special Consideration #3.)
- Pay special attention to protecting yourself from cardiovascular disease after you pass age fifty. (See Special Consideration #4.)
- Take special care of your knees, which as you'll see are constructed differently from those of men. (See Special Consideration #5.)
- To avoid back problems later in life, concentrate on strengthening the muscles of your abdomen and lower back. (See Special Consideration #6.)
- Do Achilles tendon exercises if you wear high heels. (See Special Consideration #7.)
- Condition opposing sets of muscles in different parts of the body to provide extra support and prevent injuries. (See Special Consideration #8.)
- Identify the weakest or most vulnerable parts of your body, and start now to strengthen them. (See Special Consideration #9.)
- Be aware of how exercise and a proper diet can offer protection against osteoporosis, or loss of bone mass leading to fractures in older age. (See Special Consideration #10.)

Because of the many benefits of exercise, older women are flocking in record numbers to fitness clubs and nutrition counseling organizations like our Aerobics Center in Dallas. They are also participating in a wider range of athletic activities. Many still concentrate on such fitness staples as walking, jogging, and aerobic dance. Others are plunging into weight training and competitive masters competition. Or they are returning to sports that they excelled in during their youth, such as swimming, skating, and skiing. To grasp the range of possibilities, consider the achievements of just a few of these older female athletes:

Maria Lenk Zigler, Olympic Swimmer and World Record Holder. At seventy-five years old, Maria Zigler, a Brazilian by birth, participated as a swimmer in the 1936 Olympics in Germany and at one time held the world record for women of all ages for the 200-meter and the 400-meter butterfly. She also competed regularly in masters swimming events and established several world records in older age categories.

When she came into our clinic for a complete checkup, she was in excellent health: Her blood pressure, cholesterol levels, percent of body fat, and resting and stress electrocardiogram results were typical of those of a healthy, much younger woman.

The only recommendation that I had was that she walk four to five times a week, thirty minutes a session, at a pace of fifteen minutes per mile. This mild type of weight-bearing exercise retards the loss of bone mass that is a natural part of aging. That can be especially dangerous to older women in the form of osteoporosis.

Swimming can help with this problem—especially with the bones of the arm. But there are indications that swimming may be less effective for the bones of the back and lower extremities than land-based sports. The reason: Support from the water causes less pressure on the skeletal structure than is generated by walking, jogging, or weight training. (Pressure on the skeleton causes the bone cells to become more active and generate more mass, a process that counters natural bone loss.)

Dr. Barbara Alvarez, the Iron Woman. Dr. Alvarez, who is in her early fifties, and her twin sister, Angelika Casteneda, began running when they were forty. Since that time, they have run fifty-eight marathons; finished among the top participants three times in the Ironman World Championships; and completed several ultra-marathons.

The Austrian-born pair were the only women to run in the 130-mile 1990 Marathon Des Sables in the 100-plus heat of the Sahara Desert. They had to carry twenty-three-pound knapsacks on their backs during the event. Not content with braving the African heat, the twins also turned in a top women's time of 39:27:00 in the Badwater 146, which goes through Death Valley. (See *Runner's World,* December 1990, p. 94.)

Ruth Lemke, Who Passed from Near-Death to Life. In her mid-forties, Lemke nearly died as a result of a blood clot in a lung. After that close call, she stopped smoking and started a fitness regimen. She began with walking, moved on to jogging, and finally, by age fifty-four, started racing. Not only that, she succeeded in getting her husband and six of their children to race with her in one recent event!

Sally Urban—the Return of the Skating Champ. Sally Urban and her husband, Stan, now in their late forties, won the 1963 National Ice Dancing Championships as teenagers. After they retired from competition, they got married and kept in shape by running up to thirty miles per week near their Pennsylvania home.

Then, in their forties, they decided they'd like to try ice dancing again. So they began to work on a program and suffered through the conditioning of long-unused muscles. "Our skating workouts were tough, but running definitely helped with the comeback," Sally told *Runner's World* in 1990.

The result: They won the Eastern Adult Senior Ice Dance Championships in the winter of 1990.

Many older women such as these are extending their involvement into a variety of athletic activities—and they are performing at new levels of excellence. But is rigorous exercise really good for most older women? Is it possible that too many are going too far with fitness? To answer such questions, let's first consider some of the special exercise benefits for the older female athlete.

What Can Exercise Do for the Average Older Woman?

As women age, they lose considerable amounts of muscle mass, as do men. But they usually start off with less muscle than men, and so they may deteriorate to levels of disability and poor body functioning faster than men. Consequently, because women on average live longer than men, they may have to spend extra years in a state of dependence on others, unable to wait on themselves or move about with ease. It may become impossible for them to pursue work or volunteer projects, visit friends, or engage in other activities that occupied them when they were younger.

To avoid this depressing scenario, women past about ages thirty-five to forty need to embark as early as possible on an exercise program that will ensure their continued independence. As we've already seen, the building blocks of such a program for both men and women are: 1) aerobic exercises to improve endurance, and 2) a strength/flexibility regimen to promote muscle power, suppleness, and range of motion.

THE BENEFITS OF THE PROGRAM

Such a program will have several benefits that work to the advantage of older women:

Bone loss will decrease—and the risk of osteoporosis will decline. A 1988 study involving women ages fifty-five to seventy showed that weight-bearing exercises—such as walking, jogging, and stair climbing—could actually increase bone mineral density in the lumbar (lower) spine. (We'll discuss the osteoporosis issue in more detail later in this chapter.)

Physical reaction time will improve. A study of older women at the University of Texas revealed that regular aerobic exercise can significantly improve the ability of muscles to contract and otherwise respond to stimulation.

The overall aging process will slow down. Researchers at the University of Illinois in Champaign-Urbana studied the impact of exercise on aging among 166 women, ages thirty to eighty-five. They discovered that those who exercised regularly had younger bodies, as measured by the amount of bone loss, muscle loss, and fat increase. Specifically, those of every age who were more fit had denser bones and leaner bodies than those who didn't exercise.

But in addition to these general benefits of exercise, there are also those special considerations—which I summarized at the beginning of this chapter—that older women should keep in mind as they pursue their exercise programs.

Special Considerations for the Aspiring Superwoman

SPECIAL CONSIDERATION #1: WOMEN, PERHAPS EVEN MORE THAN MEN, NEED *TOTAL* BODY CONDITIONING

This means they should have an aerobic activity *and* a strength/flexibility program. The strength/flexibility regimen is especially important to pressure muscle and bone mass in the upper body.

Note: Women do *not* have to worry about becoming muscle-bound or looking masculine if they engage in upper-body exercises, including work with weights. I recommend the use of relatively light weights with high repetitions, an approach that improves strength without emphasizing the heavy muscle development characterized by certain bodybuilding techniques.

Even if a woman does use heavier weights with lower repetitions, it's highly unlikely that she will develop a heavily muscled physique comparable to that of a male bodybuilder. The probable reason: Women lack the male hormones that produce bulky muscle development with heavy weight work.

SPECIAL CONSIDERATION #2: MOST WOMEN, LIKE MOST MEN, SHOULD LIMIT THEIR RUNNING TO NO MORE THAN TWELVE TO FIFTEEN MILES PER WEEK. AND EVEN MOST WOMEN WHO ARE INVOLVED IN COMPETITIVE RUNNING EVENTS SHOULD STAY UNDER THIRTY MILES PER WEEK

Women who are training for ultra-marathons, marathons, or other extremely long distances may want to train for longer distances each week, especially when they're conditioning themselves for a particular race. But *most* women who want to stay in superior aerobic condition—including those who are training for many of the shorter competitive events—can achieve all they need with a maximum weekly mileage of twenty-five to thirty miles.

The reason I pick this particular limit is that I've seen joint, bone, and muscle injuries increase dramatically beyond this distance. Also, female athletes who are still menstruating often find that they develop amenorrhea (a failure to menstruate) when running longer distances, in part because their body fat decreases to excessively low levels.

Those over-thirty women athletes who find they can compete effectively or otherwise stay in adequate shape with *less* than thirty miles a week should observe this general rule of thumb for fitness: There's no need to run more than twelve to fifteen miles per week to achieve optimum aerobic conditioning. Anyone who runs longer mileage should have a good reason, such as training for competitive events.

SPECIAL CONSIDERATION #3: WOMEN SHOULD TRY TO KEEP THEIR BODY FAT ABOVE 12 PERCENT BUT BELOW 22 PERCENT OF THEIR TOTAL BODY WEIGHT

Excessive body fat—above about 22 percent for women—has been associated with increased risk of heart disease. But too little body fat—below about 12 percent—may trigger amenorrhea (interruption of menstrual periods) or be associated with other health problems.

Well-conditioned women who are following a wise diet will usually have body fat in this range. If your body fat is more than 22 percent, you can get rid of the excess through a weight-loss diet or increasing the amount of your aerobic exercise. If your body fat is less than 12 percent, you should consider eating more nutritious foods, or decreasing your exercise level, or both.

SPECIAL CONSIDERATION #4: PHYSICAL PROTECTION AGAINST CARDIOVASCULAR DISEASE IS AN ACT OF *GOD* FOR WOMEN UNDER FIFTY, BUT AN ACT OF *WOMAN* FOR WOMEN OVER FIFTY

Probably to ensure the survival of sufficient numbers of females and their ability to reproduce, our Creator designed the bodies of women under fifty years of age (or those who haven't undergone menopause) with solid protection against heart disease, osteoporosis, and other serious ills. The key factor is the production by premenopausal women of estrogen, which apparently helps keep lipids, such as the "good" HDL cholesterol, elevated in the blood and affords other protections.

But the situation changes dramatically for women over fifty (or those who have gone through menopause). The protective cloak of estrogen is swept away, and women must fend for themselves. Like men, they must pay closer attention to diet, exercise, and other preventive strategies to ward off heart disease and other threats to health.

In more specific terms, about a quarter million women a year die from heart disease—about 33,000 more women than men—though the condition attacks them on average about ten years later than men. Furthermore, the main killer of women over sixty-seven is heart disease, which claims double the number of females who fall to cancer.

One 1989 study at the University of Pittsburgh, reported in *The New England Journal of Medicine,* investigated the changes in coronary risk factors that resulted after menopause in premenopausal women. Of these women, ages forty-two to fifty, those who went through menopause during a two-and-one-half-year period began to receive hormone-replacement therapy. That is, they received estrogen to replace the estrogen they lost as a result of menopause. Another group also went through menopause but received no estrogen therapy.

The women who went through menopause but weren't given estrogen experienced a decline in their "good" (HDL) cholesterol and an increase in their "bad" (LDL) cholesterol. The menopausal women who received estrogen therapy didn't experience any change in their HDL or LDL levels.

"These results suggest that a natural menopause has an unfavorable effect on lipid metabolism, which may contribute to an increase in the risk of coronary disease," the researchers said. "Hormone-replacement therapy may prevent some of these changes."

How Postmenopausal Women Can Guard Against Cardiovascular Disease It's essential for women who have gone through menopause to take steps to shore up their lost protection against heart disease. Here's a checklist that women who have gone through menopause should keep in mind to protect themselves from heart disease:

- *Consider estrogen-replacement therapy.* This treatment, which also helps prevent accelerated bone loss after menopause, provided many women with some protection from the risk factors associated with heart disease, such as low HDL cholesterol and high LDL cholesterol.

  Caution: Estrogen treatments have also been associated with an increased incidence of endometrial (womb) cancer. Consequently, estrogen is usually administered in conjunction with progesterone, which helps offset the uterine cancer risk, but the combination of hormones negates the beneficial effects of estrogen on the blood lipids. Furthermore, estrogen may not be protective against breast cancer. Some studies indicate that the combination of estrogen and progesterone may actually increase the risk of breast cancer.
- *Lower "bad" (LDL) cholesterol through a low-fat, low-cholesterol diet.* Those who can't lower their cholesterol adequately through diet should see their physicians, who may prescribe cholesterol-lowering drugs such as niacin or lovastatin. (We'll deal with this issue for both women and men in chapter 13.)
- *Pursue a regular aerobic exercise program.* See chapter 6 for details. Such a program will help raise levels of "good" (HDL) cholesterol, lower obesity, and lower risk of death from all causes.
- *Lower high blood pressure.* High blood pressure (hypertension) is a risk factor for stroke and heart disease and may be lowered through loss of weight, increase in aerobic exercise, reducing salt

and alcohol consumption, and, if necessary, through the use of antihypertensive drugs.

- *Control diabetes.* More than twice as many women as men over age forty-five suffer from diabetes, and diabetes is a major risk factor for heart disease.
- *Overcome obesity.* Elsewhere in this chapter, I've already indicated the importance of losing excess weight, but let me make the point again in a somewhat different way: Obesity is an independent risk factor for heart disease. That is, if your percent of body fat is too high (over 26 percent of body weight for women or 20.5 percent for men), your risk of having a heart attack is greater than for someone who is not overweight. For example, women who are 30 percent over their best weight are more than twice as likely to have heart disease as those who are not overweight.
- *Stop smoking.* Women who smoke are up to six times more likely than nonsmokers to have a heart attack. Smoking decreases "good" cholesterol, increases blood pressure, produces high levels of free radicals, and is associated with more rapid increase of the clogging of the arteries (atherosclerosis), which characterizes heart disease.
- *Learn to manage stress.* A failure to handle the pressure of life can increase cholesterol, blood pressure, and other risk factors linked to heart disease. Many women have successfully combatted the stress in their lives through such means as spiritual development, relaxation techniques, and regular aerobic exercise. I would suggest that you try all three of these approaches if you feel you have any trouble handling pressure.

SPECIAL CONSIDERATION #5: MOST FEMALE KNEES ARE DIFFERENT FROM THOSE OF MEN, AND EXERCISE PROGRAMS MUST BE DESIGNED WITH THIS FACT IN MIND

The function of the large muscles running along the front of the thigh (the quadriceps) is to straighten the knee. But in women, the quadriceps tend to meet the knee at a wider angle than in men. As a result, the kneecap (patella) moves laterally and may be more subject to injury.

To prevent knee injuries, women should be especially careful about overflexing the knee. In particular, they should *never* do deep knee bends, lunges that extend the forward knee beyond a perpendicular line over the foot, squat thrusts, or other squatting-type exercises or movements that might damage the knee joint. (For that matter, men should also avoid these exercises as well.)

SPECIAL CONSIDERATION #6: WOMEN SHOULD CONCENTRATE ON STRENGTHENING THE MUSCLES IN THE ABDOMEN AND LOWER BACK

Even many aerobically fit older women have relatively weak abdominal muscles. One reason is that childbirth can stretch the abdominal tissues and lead to flaccid muscles. Another reason is that most women (like most men) don't like to do calisthenics and especially don't like sit-ups or other abdominal exercises. In fact, sit-ups tend to be the exercise in a strength/flexibility routine that most people put last or omit altogether.

Why is this? Many people who have relatively unfit abdomens find that they have to strain to do a few sit-ups, and the experience is generally unpleasant. Others don't want to bother to put padding on the floor to cushion their lower backs. As a result, their backs begin to hurt before they finish their repetitions. So they stop too early, and the lack of rigor in their routine fails to improve or even maintain their abdominal fitness.

To overcome such resistance, it's necessary first to recognize how important firm abdominal muscles are. A strong, firm lower trunk—especially the abdominal area—is essential for a stable back. If the lower back isn't supported both from the rear and the front with well-conditioned muscles, strains, muscle spasms, and other lower back problems become much more likely.

There's also a biomechanical consideration when you find yourself having to lift something a little heavier than normal. It's necessary to contract or firm up abdominal muscles so that the pelvis is stabilized during lifting or twisting movements. Without the ability to harden these muscles, a woman will become much more prone to back injuries.

SPECIAL CONSIDERATION #7: WOMEN WHO OFTEN WEAR HIGH HEELS SHOULD FOCUS ON STRENGTH/FLEXIBILITY EXERCISES FOR THEIR ACHILLES TENDONS

The wearing of high heels causes the Achilles tendon (the large, rope-like tendon at the back of the heel) to become shorter and less flexible. So women who wear high heels should pay special attention to exercises that will both strength their Achilles tendons and stretch them. In particular, I'd recommend exercises like these:

Calf Raises One type of calf raise is to stand with feet flat on the floor, then stand on your toes, and finally, return to the original position with feet flat on the floor. (See chapter 7 for a description of this exercise.)

Super Calf Raises A more demanding variation of this exercise is to use weights when you raise up on your toes. (See chapter 8 for a description.)

Caution: All calf raises, and especially this second variation, should be executed slowly and deliberately, with no jerky motions. The exercise should be terminated at any sign of pain.

Achilles Tendon Stretch   Stand facing a wall, post, or similar structure, with your right foot about one and a half to two feet from the wall and your right toes pointing toward the wall. Your left foot should be placed behind the right in a stationary stride position about three to four feet from the wall.

Now place your hands flat against the wall and lean forward, keeping both heels flat on the floor. As you lean, you should feel your Achilles tendons—especially the one in the foot farthest from the wall—begin to stretch. Very gently, rock back and forth and stretch your tendons. After about ten rocking movements, switch the position of your feet and repeat the rocking movements.

SPECIAL CONSIDERATION #8: BOTH SETS OF OPPOSING MUSCLES IN THE DIFFERENT PARTS OF YOUR BODY SHOULD BE CONDITIONED

Dr. Carol Otis, assistant team physician at the University of California in Los Angeles, has discovered that female athletes and other women who work out tend to train only one muscle group, but not surrounding or opposing muscle groups. For example, runners may work on the quadriceps (the thigh muscles) but neglect the hamstrings (the muscles at the back of the leg). Both men and women may fail to strengthen opposing muscles, but because of the lighter, less-developed musculature of many women, they seem to be more vulnerable than men to injury from this source.

This flaw in training can lead to injuries for men or women because all muscles, and especially those that are used in a favorite sport, need support from surrounding tissue. A sprinter may have quite strong quadriceps but very weak hamstrings. The result: Extending the leg beyond the normal stride (as when increasing speed or beginning a sprint) may cause the muscle in the back of the leg to be pulled.

In a similar vein, those who primarily enjoy racquet sports should be sure to do exercises that increase the strength and flexibility of *both* sides of the body, as well as other surrounding tissue. Such complete training will help prevent "tennis elbow," back injuries, and other problems associated with these activities.

SPECIAL CONSIDERATION #9: WOMEN SHOULD CHOOSE *SPECIFIC* EXERCISES THAT STRENGTHEN THOSE PARTS OF THE BODY THEY FEEL ARE MOST VULNERABLE AS THEY AGE

Because I can tell you only so much through the pages of any book, you also need to do a self-analysis of your physical condition and identify possible points of weakness or vulnerability. You may be in great shape aerobically, and in many ways you may be strong and flexible. But as you examine your own body, what potential flaws can you identify? Here are some danger signals to keep in mind.

The Runner with Weak Upper-Body Muscles   I've already indicated in other contexts that a chronic problem for many older runners, even those running highly competitive or even world-class times, is to neglect upper-body exercises.

One seventy-two-year-old female runner who put in two to three miles per day, five days a week, consistently scored in the superior category on her endurance tests on the treadmill. But bone density tests showed that the bones of her arms were only 80 percent of what would be predicted for a woman her age.

The exercise prescription: She began a light-weight regimen for the upper body, as described in chapter 8. The increased muscle mass that she experienced in only four months of such activity—and the strength-training habits she has established—promise to slow down the loss of bone density in the upper body.

The Swimmer with Weak Bones   A fifty-eight-year-old woman had begun working out in a pool when she was thirty-five years old and still swam regularly an hour a day, four times a week. She seemed trim and had developed much stronger shoulder muscles than she had possessed when younger. But her wrists and forearms were naturally thin, and a bone density test showed that both in the arm bones and in the spine, her bone mass was only 88 percent of what it should have been for a women her age.

The exercise prescription: She began to walk and then to jog twice a week and also embarked on a calisthenics and light weight-training program to build up her upper body. Now after one year, she has developed such overall conditioning and strength that she is training for a triathlon.

The Right-Handed Tennis Player with an Undeveloped Left Side   A sixty-six-year-old tennis player regularly won trophies in both singles and doubles competition for her age group. But she had periodically experienced back problems and was concerned that her right arm was significantly more developed than her left.

The exercise prescription: Her physician suspected that the back problems were directly related to the uneven muscle development of her body. Consequently, he recommended a strength/flexibility program, similar to that in chapter 8, to build up *both* sides of her body and to increase her flexibility and back mobility. The result: After only three months, she began to play better tennis; her left arm started to increase in size; and her back problems disappeared. In other words, both her medical and cosmetic concerns were resolved through a well-designed exercise regimen.

The Walker with Weak Abdominal Muscles A fifty-five-year-old woman with 18 percent body fat and excellent aerobic endurance had been on a walking program for four years. Because she walked quite fast an hour a day, five days a week, she had expected her entire body to be transformed in appearance and shape. In fact, she had lost about fifteen pounds and had developed slim, muscular legs. But her stomach still protruded, almost to the same extent that it had before she began exercising.

The exercise prescription: She embarked on an upper body strength-flexibility program, with a special focus on her abdominal muscles, including challenging numbers of sit-ups, crunches, and other abdominal exercises described in chapter 8. The result: Within only three months, her abdomen became slightly flatter. Within six months, her abdomen was noticeably flatter, though there was still some protrusion.

It's possible that she's just built in such a way that boardlike flatness in the abdominal area may be an impossibility. But there's no question that the exercises, along with greater attention to posture, including walking with the abdomen tucked in, have made a major difference in her appearance.

SPECIAL CONSIDERATION #10: GUARD AGAINST OSTEOPOROSIS

In this discussion of special exercise concerns for older women, I've referred several times to osteoporosis, or the gradual deterioration of bone density that eventually results in fractures, disability, and sometimes death. I want to conclude this chapter with a further discussion of this problem and an indication of responses that may be effective.

The Older Woman Athlete and Osteoporosis It's extremely important for older women to guard against osteoporosis because this disease is much easier to prevent than to overcome. This condition can be particularly devastating for older female athletes because it limits their activity and may eventually make it impossible for them to train or compete. So no matter how accomplished an athlete you are or how superior your endurance conditioning, you should be aware of your risks for osteoporosis and adjust your training routine and lifestyle accordingly.

The Osteoporosis Risk Factors That Can't Be Controlled Personal characteristics that predispose a person toward osteoporosis include these risk factors, which *can't* be controlled:

- family history of osteoporosis
- white, northern European, or Asian ethnic background
- fair complexion
- small-boned frame
- advancing age—Those over forty are at higher risk than younger people because their bone mass has stopped increasing and steady bone loss has set in. Those over seventy are at even greater risk because of the ongoing bone loss with age.
- menopause complete—Women who have had an early menopause are at even higher risk.
- allergy to milk or other diary products, which limits the amount of calcium intake
- no children

The Osteoporosis Risk Factors That Can Be Controlled   Now here are the risk factors that *can* be controlled. Consider what you can do to change them. Avoid:

- smoking cigarettes
- drinking alcohol
- a lack of milk, cheese, or other dairy products (even though you don't have an allergy)
- a lack of weight-bearing exercise of all parts of the body
- a low percentage of body fat (less than 15 percent of total body weight)
- a cessation of menstruation as a result of excessive exercise (even though you haven't yet gone through menopause)
- eating disorders, such as bulimia or anorexia nervosa
- a diet high in animal protein (over 20 percent of daily calories), such as red meats (Such a diet seems to wash calcium out of the system.)
- adding salt to food at the table (Both pre- and postmenopausal women experience a washing-out of calcium in the urine if there is an excessive consumption of salt.)
- a strict vegetarian diet
- too much fiber in the diet
- excessive consumption of caffeine (the equivalent of three or more cups of coffee or strong tea each day)

To combat the threat of osteoporosis, you should strive to change the above risk factors in your life that can be controlled—and failure to engage in regular weight-bearing exercise is one of the most important deficiencies that you can correct.

According to a report in the December 28, 1994, issue of the *Journal of the American Medical Association,* Drs. Miriam E. Nelson, Maria A. Fiatarone, William J. Evans, and other Tufts University researchers employed high-intensity strength training with forty postmenopausal woman, ages fifty to seventy. All the women, who were sedentary and not on estrogen replacement therapy, engaged for forty-five minutes twice weekly over the course of a year in five fairly heavy muscle-building exercises. Using resistance exercise devices, they worked on their hips, knees, shoulders, back, and abdominal area.

The results? Among the twenty exercisers, there was a consistent, significant increase in hip and back bone density, muscle mass, muscle strength, dynamic balance, and overall physical activity without the use of estrogen therapy. All of these factors contribute not only to decreased risk of osteoporosis, but also to a longer, more effective, and more active life. The message is clear: As you grow older, do regular strength-enhancing exercises!

Up to this point, we've focused on the positive—on what you should *believe* about exercise. But there are also a number of false beliefs that you should be aware of, and that you should *reject* if you hope to maximize your fitness experience.

COUNTERING THE FALSE BELIEFS ABOUT FITNESS

Just as there are false beliefs and phony prophets that may threaten your faith, there are also myths that can undercut your drive to become more fit. The most effective way to counter these mistaken notions is first to identify them and then examine them in the cold, unrelenting light of truth.

Over the years, as I've listened to confused reports from some of my patients and also the misleading arguments of would-be medical gurus, I've compiled a list of the false beliefs about fitness that I hear most often. Here are some of the most common:

- It's dangerous to exercise after age forty.
- Your maximum heart rate automatically declines as you grow older.
- It's normal for blood pressure to increase significantly with age.
- Body fat goes up with age.
- Cholesterol levels aren't an important consideration for anyone after age sixty-five.
- No increase in muscle mass is possible after you pass age sixty.
- The body's aerobic capacity (the ability to process oxygen during exercise) inevitably goes down after age forty.
- There's no value to stopping smoking after age sixty-five.
- You can't stop the loss of bone mass, or build new bone after the menopause, without estrogen replacement therapy.
- You can't reverse the process of atherosclerosis (hardening or clogging of the arteries).
- Vigorous exercise after a heart attack (myocardial infarction) is dangerous.
- The functioning of the brain and nervous system deteriorates with age.

I've already referred to some of these myths; others haven't yet been mentioned, and a number of them may surprise you. In any case, it's important to evaluate all of these false beliefs critically—and compare them with the facts—before they have a chance to creep into your consciousness and begin to chip away at your motivation and confidence.

False Belief #1: It's Dangerous to Exercise after Age Forty

Fact: Tell this to Nolan Ryan, who at forty-four years of age threw his *seventh* major league no-hitter as a pitcher for the Texas Rangers. Or check with George Foreman, who, in 1994, while in his mid-forties, defeated Michael Moorer to become the world heavyweight boxing champ for the World Boxing Association and the International Boxing Federation. Or ask Ruth Leff, who at age sixty-four became a Master's race-walking champ, even though she didn't begin exercising and competing until she was fifty-four years old.

When I was in medical school in the mid-fifties, we were told that it would be dangerous for our patients to exercise vigorously or competitively after forty years of age. There's simply no support for this myth—so long as those who are continuing or beginning to exercise have regular medical clearance. Obviously, there may be some underlying physical problem that might prevent you from participating in vigorous workouts. But if you are shown to be in good health, a graduated fitness program of the type I'm advocating in this book can be launched at almost any age.

In fact, all the evidence suggests that you'll be at *greater* risk if you fail to exercise regularly. For example, a study in the *Archives of Internal Medicine* revealed that there are three common causes of falls, which often end in permanent disability or death among the elderly: hip weakness, poor balance, and taking medications. The impact of each of these factors can often be reduced or eliminated by achieving higher levels of physical fitness and improved coordination.

In gathering evidence on the value of higher levels of physical fitness, researchers at the University of California in San Francisco studied the characteristics of more than 300 men and women who had a history of falling during the previous year. The investigators discovered that the risk of falling increased as *hand reaction time* and *grip strength* decreased!

Several studies on elderly people have shown that as older people increase their muscle mass and strength with weight lifting, their grip strength improves. Also, a correlation has been demonstrated between low-impact aerobics in older women and their reaction time. The results showed that their hand reaction time, their overall fitness, their balance, and their flexibility improved as a result of the conditioning. Such studies also suggest that regular exercise will reduce the risk of falling, which is such a major problem among the elderly. (See the *Journal of Gerontology,* Vol. 46, No. 5, pp. M162–170; and the *Research Quarterly for Exercise and Sport,* Vol. 62, No. 1, pp. 61–67.)

I could also add a personal addendum to this particular myth. I used to feel that people over sixty who hadn't exercised should limit their aerobic workouts to walking. I was leery of having any of those over this age begin vigorous exercise because I feared that perhaps their bodies "just weren't up to it."

After observing regular exercisers in their sixties, seventies, and even older begin, resume, or continue quite vigorous programs, I've changed my thinking. For those who prefer walking, I say, keep at it! After all, I include walking in my own fitness program. But if you want to try something a little more physically challenging, and if your physician gives you the go-ahead, you may want to include race walking, jogging, or competitive swimming or cycling.

Follow one of the graduated programs I've outlined in chapter 7, and you'll be on your way to a demanding yet satisfying program that can pay huge dividends in well-being—at just about any age!

False Belief #2: Your Maximum Heart Rate Automatically Declines with Age

Fact: It's true that the maximum heart rate declines as a person ages—but the main reason is a lack of aerobic conditioning. Conversely, a higher maximum heart rate can be maintained by those who participate regularly in endurance exercise, such as walking, jogging, cycling, or swimming.

Why is it important to maintain a high maximum heart rate? The answer is simple: The higher your maximum rate, the greater your working capacity (the amount of work your body can perform). When you achieve a maximum rate, exhaustion soon follows. At the point of fatigue, you must either stop or at least slow down or reduce the intensity of the activity. Older people who can perform at higher physical levels almost always have a higher than predicted maximal heart rate.

Note: In the past, to find the *predicted* maximum heart rate for people being tested on treadmills at the Cooper Clinic, we used the standard formula of 220 minus the person's age. This means that a person forty years old would have a predicted maximum heart rate of 180 beats per minute, and a person seventy years old would have a predicted maximum of 150 beats per minute.

But in my work with older patients, I've discovered that this formula often doesn't work. I may *predict* that a fifty year old will have a maximum heart rate of 170. But if he's in very good shape aerobically, he may peak out on the treadmill with an *actual* maximum of 185, which is what would be predicted for a thirty-five-year-old!

In short, those who are in outstanding condition tend to have higher-than-predicted maximum heart rates. That has led me to conclude that the expected decline with age in maximum heart rates isn't inevitable. A couple of examples from our clinic illustrate this phenomenon:

THE SIXTY-SIX-YEAR-OLD MARATHONER

When this man came to our clinic fifteen years ago, his performance on the treadmill classified him in the top 5 percent of men younger than age thirty! Even though he was fifty-one at the time, his maximum heart rate was 191, compared with a predicted maximum of 169. In other words, his heart could increase to a rate that would be expected of a twenty-nine-year-old man.

But this patient didn't rest on his laurels. He continued to run competitively in long distance events and came back to the clinic regularly for examinations. When he returned at age sixty-six, his maximal heart rate had only dropped to 189. That's a loss of two beats in fifteen years. His heart was functioning at a level that would have been fitting for a thirty-one year old. In fact, he was still in the top 5 percent of fitness for men less than thirty.

My conclusion: As far as maximum heart rate and endurance capacity are concerned, this man has dramatically slowed down the aging process. His Fitness Age in these categories is about thirty, even though his chronological age is sixty-six.

THE CHAMPION WALKER, RUTH LEFF

Ruth first came to our clinic in 1981, when she was fifty-four years old. At that time, she could walk only ten minutes and twenty seconds on the treadmill before she became exhausted at a maximum heart rate of 189 beats per minute.

Granted, her maximum heart rate was higher than we would have predicted for most women her age: She should have had a maximum rate of about 166 (220 minus her age). But her endurance performance on the treadmill placed her in a relatively low category of aerobic fitness.

But then, Ruth started to work out. She walked faster and farther several days a week, and eventually she began to compete as a race walker. In fact, as I mentioned in the first chapter, she's set eight national race-walking records for women in her age category.

When Ruth returned for testing at the clinic nine years later, she proceeded to disprove a number of myths. First, she showed that beginning competitive exercise after age forty is definitely not dangerous and, in fact, can be highly beneficial.

Second, her maximum heart rate actually went *up* as she aged. In 1981, her maximum rate was 189 beats per minute; in 1990, at age sixty-three, her maximum was 195.

Third, her aerobic capacity increased dramatically. In effect, she *doubled* her heart's working capacity by walking for twenty minutes and three seconds on the treadmill, a performance that placed her in the "superior" category for women forty to forty-nine years, and in the "excellent" category for women younger than thirty.

Furthermore, in contrast to the "normal" response of adding weight as you age, Ruth lost more than ten pounds in that nine-year period, going from 121 to 110.5 pounds.

Such experiences have convinced me that the old rule of 220 minus the age for the maximum heart rate reflects an *adaptive* response, rather than a firm, physiologic one. That is, you can influence your maximum heart rate through your lifestyle. You can maintain a younger, higher-than-expected maximum rate simply by pursuing regular aerobic exercise.

Consequently, at the clinic we now use the formula 205 minus one-half the age for those who are involved in regular conditioning programs. So if a fifty-year-old man is in good condition aerobically, we predict his heart rate by subtracting 25 (one-half his age) from 205 to get 180 beats per minute. (In contrast, a nonconditioned person would have a 170 predicted rate, according to the traditional 220 minus the age calculation.)

As you can see, we still expect some decline to occur in the maximum heart rate with age. No amount of exercise will prevent that. But the magnitude of the drop can be minimized with a regular endurance program.

False Belief #3: It's Normal for Blood Pressure to Increase Significantly with Age

Fact: Another way of stating this myth is for laypeople and doctors to say, "It's normal for the systolic blood pressure (the upper or first reading) to be 100 plus your age." For example, a sixty-four-year-old woman could expect to have systolic blood pressure of 100 plus sixty-four, or 164 mm Hg. Or a forty-eight-year-old man could feel comfortable with 148 mm Hg.

Unfortunately, such ideas, which were taught and accepted for years, are incorrect and potentially dangerous. In the first place, systolic blood pressure that is above 140 at *any* age is regarded as borderline hypertension.

And a measurement above 160 is classified as full-fledged systolic hypertension. Those who consistently have blood pressure at these levels are at a
much higher risk to suffer strokes, heart attacks, and a variety of other ills.
Consequently, it's essential that those with measurements at these levels
take steps to lower their pressure.

One of the best arguments against the rise-in-blood-pressure myth is
our ongoing study of blood pressure of more than 50,000 patients at the
Cooper Clinic. Those at the median or the fiftieth percentile—that is, 50
percent are above and 50 percent are below that level—show that there
needs to be little or no change in blood pressure among those who stay fit.

Specifically, the median blood pressure reading for men under thirty
years of age was 120/78, a figure that's well within the normal range.
(Remember, anything less than 140/90 is considered normal.) The measurements rose to 120/80 for those thirty to forty-nine; crept up slightly to 125/82
for those fifty to fifty-nine; and hit a high of 132/82 for those over sixty.
Obviously, these people have completely normal blood pressure, and their
experience directly contradicts the myth that 100 plus your age for the
systolic reading should be considered normal.

The same trends are true for women. The mean for those under thirty
was 110/70. The measurement rose to 120/80 for those fifty to fifty-nine
years old, and to only 130/80 for those older than sixty.

Of course, some people are more prone than others to rises in blood
pressure with age. Dr. Norman Kaplan, the internationally recognized expert on hypertension from the University of Texas Southwestern Medical
Center in Dallas, recommends that older people try the same nondrug therapy used by younger patients. This approach includes:

- weight reduction
- restriction of sodium to two grams per day
- moderation of alcohol
- regular aerobic exercise

He notes that older people tend to be more sodium-sensitive than those
who are young. If diet or other nondrug approaches don't work, Kaplan
recommends that the patient's physician consider drug therapy. (See Jong I.
Tjoa and Norman M. Kaplan, "Treatment of Hypertension in the Elderly,"
Journal of the American Medical Association, Vol. 262, pp. 1015–1018.)

False Belief #4: Body Fat Goes Up with Age

Fact: It's true that both body fat and weight usually go up with age
in the general population. But again, this change is primarily an adaptive

response, as a result of a failure to maintain adequate muscle strength and conditioning. It's not a change that arises from some unalterable biologic or physiologic imperative.

Our records at the Cooper Clinic show that the percent of body fat of men, as measured by a combination of techniques using calipers and underwater weighing, increases from a median of 16 percent for those under age thirty to 22.6 percent for those over age sixty. For women, the median increase is 21.1 percent to 30 percent for this age range.

But these people represent a general sampling and are not limited to those who are fit. We recommend that men keep their percent of body fat between 15 and 19 percent, and for women, we prefer body fat between 18 and 22 percent. How can they maintain these levels? The answer is simple: Do regular endurance exercise; pursue a strength-building program; and restrict calories when necessary.

For example, in one of our studies, we found that men who averaged 44.5 years of age and were in the excellent fitness category had only 18.2 percent body fat. By contrast, those at the average level for the forty to forty-nine year age group had nearly 21 percent body fat.

Clearly, if a person fails to watch his diet or to pursue a regular exercise program, his percent of body fat will increase with age. But if he keeps in good shape by exercising aerobically and following a muscle-building program, his body fat measurements will increase only minimally with age.

False Belief #5: Cholesterol Levels Aren't an Important Consideration after Age Sixty-Five

Fact: Actually, we need to be concerned about high cholesterol levels at *any* age. This fact was confirmed by a January 19, 1990, article in the *Journal of the American Medical Association,* which documented elevated serum cholesterol levels as a risk factor for coronary heart disease in the elderly.

In this study, 1,480 men, age sixty-five and older, were followed for an average of twelve years. The greater incidence of deaths from heart disease in those with high cholesterol supported the argument that high cholesterol is an independent predictor of coronary heart disease, even among men over sixty-five.

A study conducted at Yale University and published in November 1994 in the *Journal of the American Medical Association* did conclude that high cholesterol had no predictive value for heart disease for people over seventy years of age. But Dr. William P. Castelli, director of the famed Framingham study of heart disease, believes that the weight of other data shows that high cholesterol is an important risk factor for men and women of any age. At this point I agree with Dr. Castelli, and I certainly continue to recommend low-fat diets, cholesterol-lowering drugs, and other measures to reduce blood lipids in older people who have a high risk profile for heart disease.

The lesson to remember is this: You're never too old to forget about your cholesterol level, and you're never too old to benefit from a reduction in cholesterol.

False Belief #6: No Increase in Muscle Mass Is Possible after Age Sixty

Fact: We've already seen in previous chapters that it *is* possible to increase muscle mass after age sixty, even though the average person tends to lose 30 to 40 percent of muscle mass during a lifetime.

How do you prevent a loss of muscle, and even increase your muscle mass in your older years? The answer is evident in a study done at the U.S. Department of Agriculture Human Nutrition Research Center on Aging at Tufts University.

In a report in the *Journal of the American Medical Association* of June 13, 1990, the Tufts researchers noted that muscle weakness and related immobility led to an increased risk of falls, fracture, and dependency. Their study concentrated on nine "frail, institutionalized" volunteers averaging ninety years of age and ranging up to ninety-six years. These participants experienced dramatic increases in strength and muscle girth as a result of an eight-week training program.

The investigators put the volunteers on a progressive resistance training program involving a weight machine. The participants performed three sets of eight repetitions with each leg. Six to nine seconds were allowed for each repetition, with one to two minutes of rest between sets. The sessions were conducted three times each week. As the participants grew stronger, the weights with which they were exercising were increased to no more than 80 percent of their one-repetition maximum load.

At the end of the eight weeks, tests revealed that the average strength gain was 174 percent. Also, their total midthigh muscle area increased by 9 percent, and their quadriceps (front thigh muscles) increased by nearly 11 percent.

Furthermore, there was a 48 percent increase in their "tandem gait speed" (ability to walk quickly). In addition, two of the participants found they no longer had to use canes to walk. One of the participants who hadn't been able to rise from a chair without the use of his arms could do so at the end of the program.

The researchers said, "We conclude that high-resistance weight training leads to significant gains in muscle strength, size, and functional mobility among frail residents of nursing homes up to ninety-six years of age."

An interesting side note: All the participants resumed their sedentary lifestyles after the training program ended, and their physical fitness went downhill again. After only four weeks of this "detraining," the group experienced a 32 percent loss of maximum strength.

False Belief #7: The Body's Aerobic Capacity (or the Ability to Process Oxygen during Exercise) Inevitably Goes Down after Age Forty

Fact: You'll recall from chapters 4 and 5 that those who engage in regular endurance exercise can maintain a high aerobic capacity from age forty to about age seventy. It's only in their seventies and eighties that older athletes usually begin to experience significant declines in aerobic ability. And even at that age those who continue to work out can remain remarkably fit.

In related investigations, Dr. Michael Pollock, who has done research at Wake Forest University, the Aerobics Center in Dallas, and the University of Florida, has studied the aerobic capacity of masters runners. He discovered that the endurance abilities of athletes forty to sixty-nine years old "were strikingly similar. There was no significant decline." (See Stu Stuller, "Run Long and Prosper," *Runner's World,* July 1986, p. 78.)

Then, Pollock did a ten-year follow-up on his original study. He found that those runners who continued to run competitively experienced no loss of aerobic capacity. In contrast, those who trained less intensely had a 9 percent loss of aerobic capacity during the ten-year period—the same decline that other studies show for sedentary people.

The lesson here is that to maintain aerobic fitness as you age, it's essential to *keep up your training intensity.* Those who work hard to retain their endurance will have a good chance to hold off this sign of aging.

An interesting addendum to Pollock's research: Both the competitive and the noncompetitive runners experienced a significant loss of lean body mass; that is, their muscle size declined and their percentage of body fat went up. The most significant exceptions were three who did upper-body strength work on a regular basis. Two of these people were on a weight-training program, and the other was a cross-country skier.

In another study, reported in April 1990 in *The Physician and Sportsmedicine,* researchers from San Diego State University came to a somewhat different conclusion as they explored the decline of aerobic power with age. Two groups participated in the study: Fifteen, who exercised regularly, were followed for twenty-three years, from age forty-five to sixty-eight. Another fifteen, who didn't exercise, were followed eighteen years from ages fifty-two to seventy.

The results: The exercisers experienced a decline of 13 percent in their aerobic capacity, while the nonexercisers experienced a 41 percent decline. The researchers ended with this observation: "The data suggest that regular aerobic exercise retards the usual loss in aerobic power with age."

The 13 percent loss in aerobic capacity among the exercisers was attributed to two common aspects of aging: 1) a lower maximal heart rate (an average drop of twenty beats per minute over the twenty-three-year period), and 2) a lower stroke volume (a measurement of the ability of the heart to pump efficiently).

I conclude from such studies that endurance capacity can be expected to decline with age. But the *rate* of that decline can be reduced with an endurance or aerobic program. Furthermore, regular endurance activity can probably *postpone* the onset of the most significant decline in endurance. In other words, a person who engages in regular aerobic workouts may not experience a significant drop in aerobic activity until his late sixties. But if he didn't work out, he would begin to lose his aerobic capacity at a much earlier age.

False Belief #8: There's No Value to Stopping Smoking after Age Sixty-Five

Fact: I constantly run into smokers in their sixties, seventies, or even eighties who tell me, "I'm going to continue smoking because the way I look at it, if the cigarettes haven't killed me by now, they'll never kill me!"

Another common excuse goes like this: "I've been smoking for so long, it wouldn't be of any value for me to quit."

In fact, continuing to smoke keeps the smoker at a high level of risk for heart disease and other health problems—regardless of age. A 1984 report in the *Journal of the American Medical Association* focused on the impact of smoking on the health of 2,674 people ages sixty-five to seventy-four. The researchers discovered that over a period of five years, those who couldn't break their habit were 52 percent more likely to have a heart attack or to die suddenly than were those who stopped smoking. A 1985 study in the same journal found that within two weeks after breaking the habit, older people experienced improved blood circulation to the brain.

These and similar results from later studies suggest that elderly people who have smoked for three or four decades aren't "lost causes." They can benefit significantly by abstaining from smoking.

False Belief #9: You Can't Stop the Loss of Bone Mass or Build New Bone after the Menopause without Estrogen Replacement Therapy

Fact: See chapters 4 and 10 for more detailed information that explodes this myth. As I've said, regular, weight-bearing exercise, along with adequate consumption of calcium and vitamin D, can help hold off the loss of bone mass associated with aging.

Note: It may also be advisable for women who have gone through menopause to undergo estrogen-replacement therapy to treat diagnosed osteoporosis. Be sure to check with your physician if you're in this category.

False Belief #10: You Can't Reverse the Process of Atherosclerosis (Hardening or Clogging of the Arteries)

Fact: Increasingly, the scientific evidence shows that atherosclerosis, the major cause of heart disease and heart attacks, *can* be reversed, either through dietary and other lifestyle changes, or by using drugs. A couple of cases in point:

REVERSAL THROUGH LIFESTYLE CHANGES

Many experts in preventive medicine have believed for years that it's possible to reverse the ravages of atherosclerosis, and several studies have supported this belief. The most definitive report to date has come from Dr. Dean Ornish and his team of researchers from the University of California at San Francisco School of Medicine.

According to a 1990 report in *The Lancet,* Ornish assigned twenty-eight patients with coronary artery disease to an experimental program involving a low-fat vegetarian diet, a no-smoking requirement, stress management training, and moderate exercise. Another group of twenty control patients with coronary artery disease were assigned to normal medical supervision.

At the end of one year, the investigators found that the average clogging of the least diseased arteries in the experimental group *regressed* from 40 percent to 37.8 percent. In contrast, in the control group, the clogging progressed from 42.7 percent to 46.1 percent.

The results were even more dramatic with arteries that were more clogged with fatty plaque. When arteries were more than 50 percent blocked off, the experimental group experienced a regression from 61.1 percent to 55.8 percent. That is, these arteries were opened up by more than 5 percent in just one year. The patients who were not on the lifestyle-change program again suffered increased progression of their disease, with artery blockages advancing from 61.7 to 64.4 percent.

The details of the program followed by the experimental group can serve as a kind of blueprint for what it takes to reverse atherosclerosis: Their diet contained about 10 percent of calories as fat, 15 to 20 percent as protein, and 70 to 75 percent as complex carbohydrates (such as fruits, vegetables, and whole grains). Cholestrol intake was limited to less than 10 milligrams per day.

The stress management techniques included stretching, breathing techniques, meditation, and various relaxation methods. Exercise involved walking for most patients at a level of intensity that raised their heart rates to a target of 50 to 80 percent of their maximum heart rates. They were asked to exercise a minimum of three hours per week and to spend a minimum of thirty minutes per session within their target heart rates.

The researchers concluded that "overall, 82 percent of experimental-group patients had an average change towards regression. Comprehensive lifestyle changes may be able to bring about regression of even severe coronary atherosclerosis after only one year, without use of lipid-lowering drugs." (Dean Ornish, et al., "Can lifestyle changes reverse coronary heart disease?" *The Lancet,* July 21, 1990, Vol. 336, pp. 129–133.)

REVERSAL THROUGH DRUGS

Sometimes lifestyle changes, such as a low-fat diet, regular exercise, and stress reduction techniques, may not be enough to reverse clogging of the arteries. In these cases, a doctor may prescribe drugs, often with great success in overcoming atherosclerosis.

A 1990 study reported in *The New England Journal of Medicine* showed the beneficial impact that can be achieved through intensive treatment with certain drugs. In this investigation, patients with coronary artery disease were assigned to three treatment groups. One took the drugs lovastatin and colestipol; the second took niacin and colestipol; and the third was given a placebo or only colestipol.

The results: The first two groups, who underwent the most aggressive drug treatment, experienced the least progression of their coronary artery disease and the most regression.

Specifically, only 21 percent of those who took lovastatin and colestipol experienced any progression in their disease. Also, 32 percent in that group enjoyed some regression or reversal of their disease. In the niacin-colestipol group, 25 percent experienced progression of their disease, and 39 percent underwent regression. In contrast, those in the third group—who took only a placebo or colestipol—46 percent suffered further progression of their disease, and only 11 percent saw any regression.

The researchers noted that the more intensive drug therapy in the first two groups "reduced the frequency of progression of coronary lesions, increased the frequency of regression, and reduced the incidence of cardiovascular events." (Greg Brown, M.D., et al., "Regression of Coronary Artery Disease as a Result of Intensive Lipid-lowering Therapy in Men with High Levels of Apolipoprotein B," *The New England Journal of Medicine,* November 8, 1990, Vol. 323, pp. 1289–98.)

This particular myth should remind *everyone* over forty—and that definitely includes those who are competitive athletes—that physical training is only part of aging successfully and vigorously. The exercise guru Jim Fixx, author of the bestseller *The Complete Book of Running* and other popular works, was an outstanding older athlete. But because he neglected regular medical checkups and other basics of good health, he died at age fifty-two of a heart attack while on a training run in Vermont in 1984.

False Belief #11: Vigorous Exercise after a Heart Attack (Myocardial Infarction) Is Dangerous

Fact: Regular, medically supervised exercise is an integral part of most cardiac rehabilitation programs. The safety of exercising as part of a monitored rehabilitation program may be greater than exercise in the general population!

A 1986 study at the Cardiac Rehabilitation Program, Alvarado Hospital Medical Center in San Diego, reported on 51,303 heart patients who exercised over a five-year period, for a total of more than 2.3 million hours. Twenty-one cardiac arrests were reported during that time (an average of one incident per 109,500 person hours of exercise). Only three died while exercising—a fact which may be a tribute to the presence of trained medical personnel at the exercise facility. By comparison, a study of Rhode Island joggers from 1975 to 1980 found that the incidence of sudden death during exercise was one per 396,000 person-hours of exercise.

The San Diego researchers concluded that patients in cardiac rehabilitation programs may be slightly more likely to experience a cardiac arrest than nonpatient joggers. But the patients may also be less likely to die due to the availability of immediate medical attention.

Our experience at the Aerobics Center in Dallas has been even more encouraging for exercisers. After 10 million miles of running, more than 1 million miles of cycling, and 122,000 miles of swimming by more than 10,000 participants, we've only had *two* reported cases of major cardiac incidents during or after exercise and only one death.

One probable reason for this safety record is a requirement we have for all members of our Aerobics Activity Center who are over forty. Men over forty and women over fifty must have a maximal performance treadmill stress electrocardiogram before becoming active members of our club. Furthermore, their membership cannot be renewed unless they are stress-tested again at least every three years, regardless of their level of fitness or physical activity.

Using this approach, we have discovered many abnormalities among people who have no symptoms. Those with serious problems that have been uncovered by stress tests include two competitive marathoners, both in their mid-fifties. The tests showed that they had severe obstructive coronary artery disease, which had developed since their last evaluation. Probably, this discovery prevented them from having a severe cardiac problem, the first symptom of which may have been sudden death.

Overall, there is only a slight chance of having a heart attack either during regular exercise *or* as part of a well-run cardiac rehabilitation program. In any event, you can minimize your risks significantly if you'll be sure to have regular annual medical checkups, including a stress electrocardiogram.

Finally, a question that may arise in some people's minds is, "Why exercise at all if there's even a *slight* risk of a heart attack or death?"

The answer is that the risks are far greater for those who don't exercise. In the first place, regular physical conditioning improves the ability of older people to function well and certainly helps prevent accidents, such as falls. Second, a study we conducted of 10,224 men and 3,120 women at the Cooper Clinic, which was reported in 1989 in the *Journal of the American Medical Association,* showed that men and women at the lowest level of physical fitness were more than twice as likely to die of all causes as persons who merely avoided inactivity.

There are risks no matter what path you choose in this life. But the risks are far lower for those who follow a wise, systematic conditioning program.

False Belief #12: The Functioning of the Brain and Nervous System Deteriorates with Age, and Exercise Can't Do a Thing to Help This Problem

Fact: Changes do occur in the brain as we age. For example, the brain loses about 10 percent of its weight, and some of its nerve cells disappear. But it's not at all clear that the older you get, the less intelligent you become. Some researchers are arguing just the opposite, and they're linking the maintenance of mental powers to good health and fitness.

Dr. Charles Emery conducted a twelve-week study at the University of California on forty-eight people whose average age was seventy-two. He had them exercise three times a week for one hour sessions consisting of rapid walking, leg lifts, and other such activities. At the same time, he gave the participants tests to assess their problem-solving abilities, emotional state, and ability to concentrate.

His findings: Increased physical fitness was linked to a decrease in emotional problems such as depression and to an improvement in the ability to remember, to concentrate, and to reason logically.

In a similar study, researchers at Scripps College in Claremont, California have reported in a study of three hundred older people, who ranged in age from fifty-five to eighty-eight, that those who exercised often could remember, reason, and solve problems better than those who didn't exercise.

There's still considerable controversy in this area because of a lack of strong studies linking fitness to mental functioning. But at this point the indications are that those in better physical shape can expect to be in better mental shape.

Dr. James Fozard, associate director of the National Institute on Aging, directs a study that began in 1958 and that has dealt with the mental abilities of older people. Fozard and his associates have found that the mental capacities of healthy older and younger people are often quite similar.

Fozard's colleague, Dr. Gene Cohen, told *The New York Times:* "Increasingly, changes that were said to be aging are now thought to be due to illness."

Many other false beliefs about fitness might be mentioned as part of this list. For example, there's a prevalent myth that says you'll lose your sex drive as you grow older. In fact, the intensity of the sex drive may lessen, but many healthy and fit men and women find that they can enjoy sex well into old age.

Another myth says that the state of your blood automatically deteriorates with age. But recent research has shown that your immunity, hemoglobin, clot-dissolving substances, and other components of blood can remain quite high among those who are healthy and physically fit.

The main point to keep in mind is that the exerciser who pursues a regular and wise conditioning program will be much more likely than the average older person to foil the myths and enjoy more energy and a longer life.

A Second Wind for Your Body and Mind

As you can see, there is sometimes a kernel of truth in many of the commonly held myths. Yet without exception, they distort the truth about the ongoing benefits of fitness. Remember, your physical potential as you age is greater than you have been led to believe.

To be sure, our bodies do begin to break down at some point. Advanced years eventually trigger a genetic limit, which we can't alter with lifestyle changes, drugs, or other medical intervention. But by rejecting the myths and seeking the real truth about your body and its capabilities, you'll find that you can go much further and perform more efficiently than you ever dreamed possible.

In effect, you can get a second wind from your body and mind if you'll just learn how to remove the power of the myths from your own life. By pursuing an intelligent physical conditioning program, committing yourself to sound nutritional habits, and enhancing your general health through such disciplines as a regular medical exam, you can postpone the aging process *and* maximize your physical potential.

One final thought: Being in top physical condition as you age may prepare you better for unexpected medical problems. One of my patients, who had been exercising for years, was diagnosed as having prostate cancer. He was completely demoralized until he discovered that the cancer was encapsulated and that there were no signs of any spread or metastasis.

There was a hitch, however. The preferred treatment if a person wants a chance for a complete cure, is surgical removal. But the standard treatment for men over seventy (he was seventy-two) is radiation, which usually delays the growth of the cancer, but isn't curative.

After his preoperative evaluation was completed, the physicians determined that his outstanding level of fitness had given him the body of a man fifteen years younger. So the decision not to operate was reversed, and successful surgery was performed.

"All these years of exercise paid off, Doc," was his comment as he returned to a full, active, and healthy life.

Despite his temporary setback with his prostate, he demonstrated that he has not only rejected the false beliefs about fitness, but he is also the kind of person who has caught a glimpse of a kind of fountain of youth—which we will be talking about in the following chapter.

13

IS THERE A FORMULA FOR THE FOUNTAIN OF YOUTH?

The reports in the book of Genesis of how people like Enosh, Methuselah, and Noah could have lived longer than nine hundred years have long puzzled Bible scholars and have caused some to wonder if maybe the ancients had access to some secret of longevity that we have lost. This idea may have inspired adventurers like Juan Ponce de León to embark on a search for a "fountain of youth," and even though they failed in their quest, the desire to turn back the clock remains alive.

We've already seen how a regular exercise program can turn back the clock and help you lower your Real Age below your chronological age. But is it really possible to add more years to your life—and to ensure that those extra years will be vigorous and productive?

To answer this question, I usually divide the desire to retard aging into two distinct objectives:

- the retention of a look and feeling of "youthfulness"
- the actual achievement of greater longevity, or a longer life

The first of these involves maintaining or recapturing the energy, vigor, strength, and youthful looks that characterize adults in their twenties, thirties, and in some cases, early forties. The second objective concerns the extension of life to the maximum number of years genetically possible for a given individual.

These two objectives are not mutually exclusive; they are linked in many respects. Getting rid of excess fat will make you look younger and at the same time will increase your chances for living longer. But keeping the twofold distinction on aging in mind will help us formulate a *total* strategy for living long and well.

The Essence of the Fountain

Medical experts often distinguish between life expectancy and life span. Life expectancy is the average number of years that a given population can expect to live from birth. Life span refers to the maximum age that one individual can live, given his or her genetic makeup.

In the United States, the average life expectancy is currently about seventy-five years—seventy-two years for men and seventy-eight years for women. Of course, not all groups in the American public have the same average life expectancy. Blacks, for example, could expect in 1989 to live a little less than seventy years on average. The discrepancy is due to a number of factors, including average poorer health among blacks and their greater vulnerability to death by homicide.

As I've said earlier, I believe that the *maximum* average life expectancy for Americans is about eighty-five years of age—eighty-two for men and eighty-eight for women. This figure assumes that the major diseases such as heart problems and cancer would be eradicated or minimized and most people could live out their full genetic potential.

It's possible, of course, that I'm being conservative with this projection. It could be that the potential average life expectancy is higher, say in the neighborhood of age ninety or above. And certainly, many individuals can live out a much longer life span, perhaps to an outside limit of 110 or 115 years—or close to the early biblical designation of 120 mentioned in Genesis 6. But at some point, no matter how fit we stay and how many diseases we conquer, mortality will take over.

In short, there are some aspects of the aging process that simply can't be changed. Each of us has a genetic predisposition to age at a certain general rate and to die within a certain range of years. Some people's hair becomes gray early, while others may see few white strands until they are in their sixties or even seventies. Other people are more likely to experience a serious health problem, such as cancer or heart disease, at a relatively early age, because of a family history of that condition. Still others may die in their nineties even though they don't "take care of themselves," while their neighbors, who are health and fitness enthusiasts, die in their mid-eighties or younger.

A Methuselah Gene?

Some have even speculated that there may be a "Methuselah gene," which virtually ensures long life (barring some unforeseen accident or other fatal mishap) for a few people. For example, some individuals have been found to have very high "good" HDL cholesterol (high density lipoproteins). Specifically, their HDLs may be measured in the range of nearly 200 mg/dl. In contrast, excellent protection for the average woman over sixty would be 75 mg/dl or above.

John Wesley's Secret Formula for a Long Life

At age eighty-five, the itinerant Anglican preacher and founder of Methodism, John Wesley, reflected in his journal on why he had enjoyed such a long and energetic life:

To what cause can I impute this, that I am as I am? First, doubtless, to the power of God, fitting me for the work to which I am called, as long as He pleases to continue me therein; and, next, subordinately to this, to the prayers of His children.
May we not imput it as inferior means,

1. *To my constant exercise and change of air?*
2. *To my never having lost a night's sleep, sick or well, at land or at sea, since I was born?*
3. *To my having slept at command so that whenever I feel myself almost worn out I call it and it comes, day or night?*
4. *To my having constantly, for about sixty years, risen at four in the morning?*
5. *To my constant preaching at five in the morning, for above fifty years?*
6. *To my having had so little pain in my life; and so little sorrow, or anxious care?*

—from Parker, Percy Livingstone, ed., *The Journal of John Wesley* (Kent, England: STL Productions), pp. 405ff.

Lessons on longevity from John Wesley:

- Make devotion and service to God a daily part of life.
- Exercise regularly.
- Sleep well.
- Manage stress effectively.

There are cases where those with such high levels of HDLs have great longevity on both the maternal and paternal sides of the family. That is, both sets of parents and grandparents lived well into their nineties or beyond. It has been suggested that those with very high HDLs and a significant family history of longevity may have a special gene that virtually assures them of long life. The genetic component for this happy aberration is thought to reside in what's known as the apo (apolipoprotein) A-I gene. The condition is known in medical terms as *hyperalphalipoproteinemia*—which I suppose is an appropriately long word for a long-life trait.

But what about those of us who haven't inherited some sort of a Methuselah gene? Fortunately, there's still plenty of hope for retaining youthfulness and attaining a long life because we can take steps to influence how we age. In other words, we can help create our own fountains of youth.

Creating Your Own Fountain of Youth

In a nutshell, there are three main factors that affect aging, both in the sense of the way we look and feel and the length of time we can expect to live. These three, which we'll explore in more detail later in this chapter, are:

- *Smoking*—those who don't smoke live longer and look younger; those who do die earlier and age faster.
- *Sedentary living*—those who are active and pursue a regular endurance and strength/flexibility program are functionally younger and live longer than those who don't.
- *Obesity*—those carrying around excess body fat look and feel older and are more likely to die younger than those who maintain their ideal weight.

In addition to the "big three," there are other important health considerations that affect youthfulness and longevity. There have been reports that certain drugs or hormone treatments, such as the human growth hormone, may promote longer life and retard the aging process. To bring you up to date on this point, I've included a section specifically devoted to drugs.

In any discussion of longevity, it's also necessary to remember the importance of reducing the risk for such major diseases as cardiovascular problems and cancer. Although we've covered these dangers elsewhere, I'll provide some special longevity-related information on this issue.

Let's take a closer look at how smoking can make anyone older, no matter how good his or her genes are.

Don't Allow Your Life to Go Up in Smoke!

So much has been said about the evils of smoking that one wonders if the public will finally become tired of the subject and say, "We already know that. Tell us something new!" Yet as long as so many continue to smoke, the message must be reiterated: If you continue to puff away, you'll look older *and* most likely you'll die younger.

Consider first the issue of youthfulness:

- Chronic lung disease, such as emphysema, which severely limits physical activity, is more common in smokers than in nonsmokers.
- Depression has been shown to be more prevalent among elderly smokers (sixty-five years of age and older) than among nonsmokers.
- Elderly smokers are more like than nonsmokers to consume excessive alcohol.
- Elderly smokers are more likely than nonsmokers to perceive themselves as less healthy.
- Smokers are more inclined than nonsmokers to get face wrinkles.

A 1991 investigation at the University of Utah Health Sciences Center studied 109 smokers and twenty-three lifetime nonsmokers. All the participants were between the ages of thirty-five and fifty-nine. The researchers discovered, after eliminating the influence of sun exposure, age, and sex, that premature wrinkling increased with cigarette use. Specifically, those who had smoked the equivalent of a pack a day for five years were almost five times as likely to have excessive skin wrinkling as nonsmokers.

Several possible mechanisms were suggested for the increased wrinkling with smoking: 1) Chemicals in smoke may activate enzymes that can damage the elastin and collagen, which keep the skin firm and wrinkle-free. 2) Substances in cigarette smoke reduce blood flow to the skin on the face and thus limit the skin's ability to repair itself. 3) Eye irritation from smoking may cause squinting, which in turn may result in wrinkling. 4) Cigarette smoking increases the level of free radicals in the body, a prominent factor in skin aging.

As for the life-threatening dimensions of smoking, the facts are clear and have been for many years. The U.S. Surgeon General Antonia Novello reported in 1990 that both men and women who smoke have a much greater chance of dying in the next fifteen years than do nonsmokers. Those who quit smoking before age fifty have half the risk of dying in the next fifteen years as those who continue to smoke.

But it's not necessary to quit young in order to benefit. People older than fifty who stop can significantly increase their chances for a longer life, according to Dr. Novello. A man age sixty to sixty-four who smokes one pack of cigarettes a day can decrease his risk of dying in the next fifteen years by 10 percent—*if* he quits.

In a similar vein, a 1991 report from the University of Utah revealed that no matter how long a person has smoked, there are great benefits to giving it up, both for men and women. Male smokers over seventy-five can expect a 20 percent higher death rate than nonsmokers. Most of the smoking deaths come from heart disease and cancer.

Despite the overwhelming evidence, fifty million Americans still smoke, and many millions more in other countries continue with the habit. They are not just harming themselves; they are also endangering those about them. The Environmental Protection Agency has reported that secondhand cigarette smoke kills 53,000 nonsmokers a year, including 37,000 from heart disease.

So if you are a smoker—or if you live with one—you can expect to age more rapidly and die sooner than those who live in a smoke-free environment.

Our own research at the Institute for Aerobics Research has shown that, without question, the totally inactive "never-smoker" has a lower risk of dying from all causes than does the regular exerciser who continues to smoke cigarettes. Regular physical activity can help to reduce the detrimental effects of many of the common risk factors, such as elevated cholesterol or high blood pressure, but exercise can't completely negate the harmful effects of smoking.

Note: Cigarette smoking is probably the worst health hazard in the world today; so the message is loud and clear: Stop now if you hope to find your personal fountain of youth.

Exercise Your Right to Longevity

A regular exercise program should be the centerpiece of any quest for youthfulness and a longer life. Physical activity can delay the process of aging and make you look and feel younger in a number of ways:

- You'll be less likely to become obese—a condition that is often associated with aging.
- Your body will stay firmer and trimmer.
- Your energy levels will be higher.
- You will have an enhanced feeling of well-being.

There is solid evidence that physically active people live longer. Our landmark study at the Cooper Clinic in Dallas, which was published in the *Journal of the American Medical Association,* investigated the relationship between fitness levels and risk of dying in more than 10,000 men and 3,000 women. The report showed that men and women with low levels of physical fitness had more than twice the mortality rate of persons with even a moderate level of physical fitness. Fitness helped overcome *all* causes of mortality, including diabetes, cancer, and heart disease.

What does it take to be fit enough to increase the chances you'll live longer? The minimum amount of exercise needed to achieve health and longevity can be summed up this way:

- *For women:* Walk two miles in less than thirty minutes three days per week. Or walk two miles in forty minutes, five days per week.
- *For men:* Walk two miles in less than twenty-seven minutes three days per week. Or walk two miles in thirty-five minutes, five times per week.

Those who exercise for aerobic fitness, not only for health and longevity, enjoy an even lower risk of an early demise. Here is a sample of the amount of exercise that will afford the *greatest* protection from all types of mortality:

- *For women:* Walk two miles in less than thirty minutes six days per week. Or run two miles in less than twenty-four minutes, four days per week.
- *For men:* Walk three miles in less than forty-five minutes, five days per week. Or run two miles in less than twenty minutes, four days per week.

Our findings are the culmination of a long line of studies that have been pointing to the benefits of exercise for a richer and longer life. For example, the famous Paffenbarger study of 16,000 Harvard alumni showed through questionnaire surveys that moderate physical exercise can increase longevity by 2.4 years. Our study was different and of even greater scientific interest since we actually measured the fitness of our subjects through treadmill stress testing and followed them prospectively for an average of 8.2 years.

Other studies have continued to add weight to the importance of exercise as a means to delay aging and lengthen life. For example, a 1991 report in the British medical journal *The Lancet* showed that people with moderately high blood pressure could reduce their hypertension with exercise alone. Antihypertensive drugs were not required. High blood pressure is a major risk factor in stroke and other cardiovascular disease.

Regular exercise is an essential source of longevity and youthfulness. So be happy that as an active exerciser you're laying a solid physical foundation for your later years.

The Fat Factor

The third major element in accelerating aging and reducing the length of life—after smoking and a lack of exercise—is what might be called the "fat factor." The fat factor refers to an excess amount of fat on any man or woman, which causes the condition known as obesity. Obesity, in short, is an excessive percent of body fat in relation to total body weight.

Women under age forty should have less than 22 percent body fat; men under forty should have less than 19 percent. Over forty, 26 percent is maximum for women and 20.5 percent is maximum for men. Any amounts of fat above these levels are excessive and accelerate the aging process, as well as increase the risk for adult-onset diabetes, hypertension (high blood pressure), and certain types of cancer.

The impact of obesity on one's appearance is obvious. Those who are fatter tend to look older than those who are leaner, trimmer, and better muscled. I was amazed the other day to encounter a forty-five-year-old woman I hadn't seen in about a year. She had put on at least twenty pounds in the interim. As a result of her increase in body fat, she looked at least ten years older than when I had last seen her.

The reverse is also true. I'm reminded of a sixty-year-old man who had been thirty-five pounds overweight, but over the course of ten months had lost the excess poundage. In addition, he had embarked on a regular aerobic and strength/flexibility conditioning program. By the end of the ten months, he appeared to be at least ten years younger.

This change in looks isn't merely a superficial transformation of the surface. People who carry around less weight both look and act younger. They are uniformly more energetic and active than those who are obese. They tend to have healthier results on their medical exams, with lower blood pressure and cholesterol levels, among other things. There are exceptions to these generalizations. But staying at your ideal weight, neither too fat nor too thin, will promote better health and a longer life.

The medical literature tends to support these conclusions. Dr. JoAnn E. Manson and other researchers, in a 1987 article in the *Journal of the American Medical Association,* surveyed the major medical studies on obesity and longevity. They said that these investigations suggest that if you weigh 10 percent less than the average American of your height and build, you'll live longer than average.

What about Subnutrition?

There are also indications from animal studies that a program of calorie restriction, or "subnutrition" as it's sometimes called, can promote dramatic increases in longevity. The problem with trying to transpose these findings to humans is that the food restriction, which in some cases doubled the life span of rats, also led to retardation of growth in the animals. That result wouldn't be desirable for humans.

But if the calories are restricted *after* growth is completed, that would be more acceptable. Some of the animal studies have shown that restricting calories after weaning or in early adulthood results in significantly improved responses of the immune systems and other benefits associated with a delay of the aging process.

So should human beings try restricting their calories in an effort to live longer? Dr. Roy Walford, a medical researcher at the University of California, has done studies that show the lives of both fish and mice can be extended through undernutrition. Walford is only one of the investigators who has discovered that restricting calories can even lengthen the life of adult animals. Walford has become so convinced by his research that he has cut far back on his own calorie consumption.

SUMMING UP SUBNUTRITION

At this point, definitive studies are lacking in showing the impact of subnutrition on life span, and so I wouldn't recommend that most people follow Walford's lead. On the other hand, there are some benefits from modified calorie restriction. I would sum up what we know about the subject this way:

- Most Americans can afford to cut back on their calories because far to many of us are carrying around excess weight.
- It's unwise to reduce calorie consumption below 1200 to 1500 calories a day unless you're on a specific, balanced weight-loss program. Even with a reduction regimen, daily calories should not go below 1200 unless you're being supervised by a physician.

Note: For athletic men and women, especially those who are in training for competitive events, a much higher intake of calories will be necessary to meet the demands of intense exercise. Each individual will have to experiment to determine what calorie level will enable him or her to maintain an ideal weight and achieve peak performance.

- Experiments in applying subnutrition to animals, as well as Dr. Walford's experiments on himself, have involved the intake of extra vitamins, minerals, and other supplements to be sure that malnutrition doesn't occur. The theory we're talking about is *sub*nutrition, or eating significantly fewer calories than you're accustomed to eating, *not mal*nutrition.
- Any reduction in weight as a result of cutting calories should not reduce a woman's percent of body fat below about 12 percent, nor a man's below about 7 percent. Athletic men may keep their percent of body fat in the range of 7 to 15 percent and athletic women at 12 to 18 percent.
- A reduction in calories should not result in chronic fatigue or low energy levels. If such a condition persists, you're probably eating too little and should increase your food intake.

Even though subnutrition can be shown to apply in some ways to animals, this approach hasn't been established as appropriate for humans. But I am open to a *modified* restriction of calories—to 1500 calories a day or another level that enables the individual to maintain an ideal percent of body fat and high levels of energy.

Can Drugs Fortify the Fountain?

Just as some young athletes have used dangerous anabolic steroids to enhance their athletic performance, older athletes are becoming increasingly fascinated by the possibility of "magic bullets" to hold off the aging process.

Young people who have relied on drugs to improve their sports abilities have paid a heavy price, with increased incidence of cardiovascular disease, cancer, and other serious health problems. Older athletes likewise face dangers with unproven fountain-of-youth drugs. So at the present time, stay away from them unless the medications are administered under the strict supervision of qualified medical personnel.

It's important for older people to keep abreast of recent advances in this area because in some instances a physician may determine that a certain drug is appropriate for a given individual. One of the substances currently being tested for its effects on aging is human growth hormone, the glandular secretion that affects the body's growth and cell reproduction.

In a July 5, 1990, report in *The New England Journal of Medicine,* Dr. Daniel Rudman and a number of other physicians and researchers studied twenty-one healthy men, ages sixty-one to eighty-one, who had become deficient in human growth hormone. (A characteristic of advancing age is the declining activity of this hormone, which may result in a lowering of lean body mass and increase in fatty tissue.)

In the study, twelve of the men received doses of human growth hormone over a six-month period, and the other nine did not. The results: In the group that received the hormone, there was an 8.8 percent increase in lean body mass; a 14.4 percent decrease in fatty tissue; and a ⅙ percent increase in average lower-back spinal mass. The group that didn't receive the hormone experienced no significant changes in these areas.

This study is only a preliminary indication of what may be possible with human growth hormone. The long-term effects on those who take it aren't clear, and caution must be exercised. In children, for instance, the drug may cause enlargement of the heart and leukemia. Also, adults who produce too much of the hormone are at higher risk for diabetes, arthritis, and excessive enlargement of the bones (acromegaly).

Indeed, a physician commenting on the above study in *The New England Journal of Medicine* concludes, "Because there are so many unanswered questions about the use of growth hormone in the elderly and in adults with growth hormone deficiency, its general use now or in the immediate future is not justified."

Still, this initial probe into human growth hormone is encouraging and tantalizing. It may be that, at some point in the future, low doses of human growth hormone will be used more generally to supplement the loss of this substance in the elderly and to enhance their muscle development and overall physical functioning.

Other drug treatments have also been suggested to retard aging or prolong life. They include deprenyl, an antidepressant that some say increases the sex drive; RU-486, the controversial French pill that induces abortions (and has been reported as a help to those with Alzheimer's disease, Cushing's syndrome, and breast cancer); and DHEA (dehydroepiandrosterone), a steroid which is found naturally in young adults but which declines with aging.

My advice on these and other unproved treatments to retard aging is unequivocal: *Stay away from them!*

At a future point, some drug may be proven to have some beneficial effects against aging without significant side effects. Currently, the anti-aging drugs and hormones are at best in the early stages of testing, either on humans or animals, and often the short- and long-term side effects are unknown. It's much better to stick with a *natural* age-combatting program, including a well-rounded regimen of exercise and good nutrition, than to take any chances with drugs that may very well backfire and cause more problems with your health than they resolve.

No discussion about finding a personal fountain of youth would be complete without a reminder about the importance of guarding against cardiovascular disease, including heart attacks and strokes, and also cancer. These threats are the main causes of death among older people, and no one can expect to live out his full life span unless he lowers the relevant risk factors.

We've already considered many of the major strategies to combat these diseases, such as having a regular medical exam, and guarding against the "big three" threats to a long life—smoking, obesity, and sedentary living. Now, let's turn to the final major component of an active, healthy, and long life: good nutrition.

Part Four

From Physical to Spiritual Food

14

INNER FOOD

Too often, those of us who live in the well-to-do Western culture take our food for granted. We always assume that a square meal will be there when we need it, and if we say a blessing before we eat, it's often a perfunctory utterance that doesn't express any deep, heartfelt thanks.

I'm all for saying blessings at meals; I always pray before I eat, whether at home, in restaurants, or in the office. But I've also come to believe that it's important for us to pray about our food and diet before we ever reach the table. I'm talking about a kind of "pre-blessing," which involves a focus on our strategy of eating and our selection of certain foods. So instead of just saying, "Lord, please bless this food to my body's use," it may be more appropriate to pray, "Please help me to choose the items and method of preparation that are going to promote good health."

I often wonder if Jesus didn't use striking nutritional images—such as calling himself the "bread of life," or offering "living water"—because he knew there is an intimate connection between the work of food in our bodies and the work of the Holy Spirit in our souls. Food, after all, is a gift from God, even if we don't always recognize that fact.

We only have to look around the world at this very moment to see how many millions are either starving or suffering from some degree of malnutrition. Our abundance—which is a very unusual phenomenon in this day and age—shouldn't blind us to the fact that God has blessed us and wants us to use his gifts in the most beneficial and healthful way possible. If we abuse our bodies with the wrong kinds of foods, we are also abusing our trust as stewards of an important part of his creation.

But because we have so much to eat, it's easy to overlook the importance of being thankful and the best way to make use of our meals. It's our own loss that we forget the spiritual, "inner" nature of the physical stuff that we take into our bodies every day of our lives. One otherwise fit and

---

Ben Franklin on Food and Drink

Benjamin Franklin peppered his *Poor Richard's Almanack* with a number of pithy say-
ings about food. Here are a few that you may even want to memorize—and recall when
you are designing your own eating program or sitting down to a meal:

Eat to live and not live to eat.

Drink does not drown Care, but waters it, and makes it grow fast.

Three good meals a day is bad living.

Wish not so much to live long as to live well.

—from Benjamin Franklin, *Poor Richard—An Almanack*
(New York: David McKay Company, Inc., 1976), pp. 60, 61, 85.

---

happy couple almost discovered too late that this sort of oversight can make
us vulnerable to major threats to health, or even life.

Blindsided by Exercise

A husband and wife, both in their sixties, had been quite active athletes for decades. He was a competitive runner who had performed well in
many distance races. She was a swimmer, cyclist, and runner who had
completed a couple of triathlons.

But the tragedy struck when she had a bicycle accident and broke her
hip and arm. He elected to spend most of his time waiting on her, and as a
result, he completely gave up on his exercise program. The physician attending them became concerned because the woman's broken bones failed to
heal properly. He noticed that the husband seemed generally depressed, and
his physical condition deteriorated noticeably. In many conversations, he
was less alert and articulate than he had been just a few months earlier.

The months dragged on, and the hip still didn't mend well enough to
allow the woman to walk by herself. Both she and her husband seemed to
have aged ten years. They were actually on the verge of becoming feeble.

The doctor identified what he thought might be the underlying cause
of the couple's problem. During a conversation with the husband, he asked
as an aside how they were eating, since the wife was normally the cook and
couldn't move around well.

"Oh, I throw things together," the husband said.

"What kind of things?" the doctor asked.

"Sandwiches, things like that."

As it turned out, this husband and wife hadn't had more than a
half-dozen hot meals in the past six months, and they almost never had

fruits or vegetables. So the doctor arranged to have a nutritionist check out the situation. She reported back that a preliminary analysis of their eating showed they weren't eating enough calories, nor were they getting necessary vitamins and minerals.

The physician immediately concluded that the problems with the healing of the wife's broken bones must be related, at least in part, to her poor eating habits. The husband's depression and loss of mental functioning also were most likely connected in part to the lack of good nutrition.

After conveying his concerns to both the husband and wife, the doctor arranged to have food sent over to them through a Meals-on-Wheels program. This new eating program worked wonders. Within only a week or two, the mood of the couple and the mental abilities of the husband improved. After only another month or two, the knitting of the wife's broken bones was almost complete.

The experience of this husband and wife is just a more dramatic example of a common problem faced by the majority of older adults, even those on regular exercise programs. That's the problem of improper nutrition. There's no point in designing and pursuing a sophisticated exercise program if you don't eat well! Good nutrition is an absolute prerequisite to building up the endurance and muscle power that will enable you to perform at your peak and function independently well into old age.

A Plan for Nutritional Priorities

It's not that most adults in our culture don't have the money or opportunity to prepare and eat the right kinds of food. The problem is often that they haven't sorted out their nutritional priorities. In effect, they become confused with the barrage of information that comes out almost daily about what you should or shouldn't eat to stay healthy. Those who are living alone may lose interest in eating, and the discipline of maintaining a regular program of good nutrition may disappear.

In this chapter, I want to help you set some simple but very important nutritional priorities. I'm not going to suggest any menus or recipes. You can find those in my other books, such as *Antioxidant Revolution*. But I am going to clarify the major issues you should keep at the front of your mind as you consider the best eating plan for your needs.

THE FOUR MAIN NUTRITIONAL ISSUES

Four basic nutritional concerns should control your grocery shopping and food preparation. These are:

Wesley In Withdrawal?

John Wesley, the Anglican preacher who founded the Methodist movement in England, made this entry in his journal on July 6, 1746:

After talking largely with both the men and women leaders, we agreed it would prevent great expense, as well of health as of time and money, if the poorer people of our society could be persuaded to leave off drinking of tea. We resolved ourselves to begin and set the example. I expected some difficulty in breaking off a custom of six-and-twenty years' standing. And, accordingly, the three first days my head ached more or less all day long, and I was half asleep from morning till night. The third day, on Wednesday, in the afternoon, my memory failed almost entirely. In the evening I sought my remedy in prayer. On Thursday morning my headache was gone. My memory was as strong as ever. And I have found no inconvenience, but a sensible benefit in several respects, from that day to this.

—from Parker, Percy Livingstone, ed., *The Journal of John Wesley* (Kent, England: STL Productions), pp. 146–147.

Lessons on inner food and drink from Wesley:

• Strictly limit or eliminate your intake of caffeine—whether tea, coffee, chocolate, or soft drinks. Caffeine causes physical dependence and in excess may well be harmful to your health.
• If you decide to go off caffeine, do so gradually. Otherwise, you're likely to experience the "withdrawal" symptoms that plagued Wesley.
• Always approach decisions and difficulties involving food or drink in an attitude of prayer—as Wesley did in asking for divine help to overcome his withdrawal symptoms. As ordinary and even trivial as the subject of diet may seem, the food you eat and the liquids you drink are a proper subject for prayer. After all, they can play a major role in your spiritual and emotional life and may be decisive in determining how well and energetic you feel—and how effectively you are able to accomplish your daily tasks.

1.   the fat-cholesterol issue
2.   the fiber issue
3.   the calcium issue
4.   the supplement issue

It's essential to understand the basics about each of the issues and then act on your knowledge. If you just keep the "big four" in mind, you'll continue to do well with your overall fitness efforts.

#1: THE FAT-CHOLESTEROL ISSUE

A major objective should be to keep your consumption of fats (especially saturated fats) and cholesterol as low as possible. The reason: The more saturated fat you consume, the higher the risk of developing elevated cholesterol, colon cancer, and other diseases. Also, there are more calories in each gram of fat (nine calories) than in each gram of protein or carbohydrate (four calories). This means that those who eat more fat are likely to become more obese.

The balance of fat, protein, and carbohydrate should generally follow the guidelines of the American Heart Association:

- no more than twenty to thirty percent of daily calories from fat
- about fifty to seventy percent of calories from complex carbohydrates (such as fruits, vegetables, legumes, and whole grain products—*not* candies, desserts, or simple sugars, which are classified as simple carbohydrates)
- about ten to twenty percent of calories each day from protein sources (such as fish, poultry, or meats)

I would go even further than the AHA guidelines. I believe it's best for the average person past thirty to design the daily diet so that the percentage of calories from fat is no more than twenty to twenty-five percent of total calories. So if you typically take in 2,000 calories per day, a maximum of 400 to 500 of those calories should come from fats.

Note: There are three types of fat—saturated, polyunsaturated, and monounsaturated. It's best to divide your daily consumption of fat into thirds, with one-third of your calories coming from each type of fat. Certain studies indicate that monounsaturated and polyunsaturated fats may help control blood cholesterol levels. But saturated fats—which generally come from animal products and can be identified because they tend to be solid rather than liquid at room temperature—*definitely* raise blood cholesterol levels and should be avoided whenever possible.

Here are some examples of foods that fit into the different fat categories: Olive oil, which derives all of its calories from fat, contains a high percentage of monounsaturated fat. Butter, also all fat, is mostly saturated fat. Corn oil, which is all fat, is mostly polyunsaturated fat.

Those with cholesterol readings above 200 mg/dl should keep their total fat below 20 percent of daily calories. It's advisable to go as low as 10 percent if cholesterol levels are above 240 mg/dl. As the percentage of calories from fat goes down, the percentage from complex carbohydrates (not from protein) should go up.

As for cholesterol, the American Heart Association suggests this rule of thumb: Daily consumption of cholesterol in foods should be 300 milligrams or less for those without blood cholesterol problems. This includes those with total cholesterol below 200 mg/dl and with a ratio of total cholesterol to HDL cholesterol of 4.5 or below for men and 4.0 or below for women.

Those who have trouble lowering their blood cholesterol level below 200 mg/dl on this diet during an eight-week trial period should reduce their dietary cholesterol consumption to below 200 milligrams per day. Those who

Will Durant on Good Nutrition

The acclaimed historian, Will Durant, who died in 1981 in his ninety-sixth year, continued to work and write with his wife, Ariel, right up to the close of his life. He had deep political and personal convictions, which included a lifelong commitment to vegetarianism—a habit that was almost certainly a major factor contributing to his long and productive life.

Here is one recollection he recorded in his journal in 1928 when he was forty-four, concerning his commitment to vegetarianism:

After barnstorming through Michigan I found myself scheduled to address the last of the teachers' convocations, October 30, in the auditorium of the Battle Creek Sanitarium—the crown and throne of the man who, more than any other since Father Mooney, had influenced my life. The American Medical Association will be amused to hear me call Dr. John Harvey Kellogg a saint of science. Most physicians, until recently, thought him a quack, a money-making charlatan. On the contrary, he was a man dedicated to spreading knowledge and health. . . .

He believed that the best way to keep the doctors away was a combination of vegetarian diet (vegetables, whole-wheat products, fruits, nuts) regular elimination, vigorous exercise, and a daily bath. He thought that meat-eating was the chief cause of disease. He did not admit that meat was necessary for physical strength; consider the bull and the horse, and had not the vegetarian Milo of Crotona, six times victor in the Olympian games, been renowned for his strength? . . .

In any case I was glad to receive an invitation from Dr. Kellogg to come and let him look at me. I found him lovable at first sight: a short, slightly stout man . . . with kindly blue eyes. . . . He was delighted to learn that I had been a vegetarian since the age of eighteen, barring my seminary days and incidental transgressions. He offered advice on almost every part of me . . . warned me against the chicken-potatoes-peas-salad-ice-cream usually provided at lecture-consuming clubs. Long before the Americans heard of cholesterol he frowned upon the use of whole milk, and its derivatives, by adults. A hundred of his recommendations—whole-wheat products, vegetable proteins, physiotherapy, hydrotherapy—have won their way into our common life. He lived—on one lung—to the age of ninety-three.

—from Will & Ariel Durant, *A Dual Autobiography*
(New York: Simon and Schuster, 1977), pp. 130, 131, 403.

Lessons on eating from Will Durant:

- A heavy emphasis on fruits and vegetables in your diet will indeed be a major source of good health. The fiber, antioxidants, and other nutrients should help you combat disease and perhaps even live a longer life.
- A *long-term* commitment to a healthy diet, high in complex carbohydrates like fruits and vegetables, is essential. Good eating brings you benefits not overnight, but over time—as both Will Durant and his doctor discovered.

still have problems getting their cholesterol down to a healthy level should go on an even stricter diet, which includes no more than 100 milligrams of cholesterol per day.

The simple message, then, is lower your consumption of fats (especially saturated fats) and your consumption of cholesterol. How can you know which food to eat and which to avoid as you design your daily menus? There are two simple rules of thumb that I recommend:

1. Whenever possible, rely on the nutritional information on food packages. These easy-to-read charts will usually tell you how many calories come from fat, and they may break down the fat into monounsaturated, polyunsaturated, and saturated. Always select products that are relatively low in saturated fat.

2. With foods that *don't* have specific nutritional information, keep these points in mind: Vegetables and fruits are generally safe because they are fat-free. But stay away from foods containing palm and coconut oil, which are high in saturated fat.

Beef and pork have relatively high amounts of saturated fat, so eat them sparingly, if at all. The white meat of chicken, turkey, and other poultry is generally low in fat, so long as the skin is removed and the food preparation is low-fat (e.g., broiled, not fried).

Fish, prepared in a low-fat fashion, tends to be low in most fats, and deepwater fish like tuna and salmon contain extra amounts of the omega-3 fatty acids, which are regarded as protective against heart disease. Shellfish generally tend to be low in fat, but high in cholesterol.

Regular cheese and dairy products, such as whole milk, are high in saturated fat, but low-fat dairy products are widely available and can provide the same nutritional value without the extra fat.

Those who want more information and charts on fats and cholesterol should consult my book *Controlling Cholesterol* (Bantam, 1989).

#2: THE FIBER ISSUE

One way to be sure that you eat less fat and cholesterol is to increase your consumption of foods that are high in fiber. In general, this includes fruits, vegetables, whole-grain products, and cereals that contain plenty of fiber. By eating such foods, you'll automatically eat a higher percentage of complex carbohydrates and a lower percentage of fat, including saturated fat.

As part of the fat-reduction process, fiber provides a number of important health benefits:

The Cholesterol Benefit Certain fibers—known as soluble fibers because they dissolve in water—have been shown to help reduce the level of cholesterol in the blood. In particular, oat bran and oatmeal have been linked in various studies to a reduction of cholesterol.

In contrast to these findings, one study by Janis Swain and other researchers from the Harvard Medical School, published in the *New England Journal of Medicine* (Jan. 18, 1990), argued that oat bran has little cholesterol-lowering effect. The researchers concluded that high-fiber and low-fiber dietary grain supplements reduce serum cholesterol levels about equally simply because they replace dietary fats.

But there are several problems with generalizing too much from this study. The participants had very low cholesterol when they began their participation in the study. You wouldn't expect much of a change with such people. Also, oat bran maintained or raised levels of HDL ("good") cholesterol. But the low-fiber diet lowered the levels of HDL, not at all a desirable result.

My conclusion from this controversy is that it's still wise for the average person to continue to include significant amounts of soluble fiber in the diet. This would include oat bran, oatmeal, and dried beans.

The Colon Benefit   Another type of fiber, known as insoluble fiber because it doesn't dissolve in water, has been linked to important health advantages, including these:

- it acts as a laxative to promote easier and more frequent bowel movements
- it has been associated with prevention of colon cancer

No one quite understands why insoluble fiber should help prevent cancer of the large intestine, but a number of possible explanations have been offered. For example, one reason might be that fiber helps reduce the transit time of the stool in the intestines and thus gives carcinogens (cancer-producing substances) less time to do their work. Or there may be some substances in the fiber itself that bind the cancer-causing substances.

Foods that have high amounts of insoluble fiber include those with much wheat bran (such as All-Bran, whole wheat bread, and whole wheat spaghetti), and vegetables, such as broccoli and raw cabbage. The so-called cruciferous vegetables have been linked to a lower incidence of colon cancer and other gastrointestinal cancers. These include the "two B's" and "two C's"—broccoli, Brussels sprouts, cauliflower, and cabbage. And foods such as spinach and collard greens may protect against macular degeneration, a major cause of blindness for Americans over sixty-five years of age.

#3: THE CALCIUM ISSUE

Because bone loss becomes an increasing concern as a person ages, it's important to take every possible *natural* step to preserve bone mass. We've already seen in chapters 7 and 11 how exercise can help promote stronger, tougher bones. But nutrition—especially the intake of calcium—is also an extremely important factor. In particular, women who are prone to osteoporosis should pay very close attention to their daily consumption of calcium. (See the discussion on osteoporosis in chapter 11.)

The Recommended Dietary Allowance (RDA) for calcium is 800 milligrams per day, but I prefer that my patients stay in the 1000 to 1500 milligrams range. That's the amount endorsed by the National Institutes of Health. A higher consumption of calcium is particularly important for older people who are in the process of losing bone mass simply as a result of the aging process. Our bone mass peaks somewhere between ages twenty-five and forty, and then there is a steady decrease in bone as we get older. Exercise and high calcium intake can help retard this process.

Foods that contain relatively high amounts of calcium include: skim milk (one eight-ounce glass = 300 mg); lowfat, plain yogurt (one cup = 415 mg); part-skim ricotta cheese (½ cup = 340 mg); salmon (three ounces = 170 mg); collards (one-half cup = 180 mg); and broccoli (one-half cup = 100 mg).

A note on lactose intolerance: Aging causes many people to have deficient amounts of an enzyme called *lactase* which helps the person digest a milk sugar known as *lactose*. Without enough lactase, a "lactose intolerance" develops, with the result that eating dairy products may trigger diarrhea, gas, cramps, or other discomforts.

But it's important to understand that lactose intolerance is not an "either-or" condition; in other words, you don't necessarily have a bad case of it or avoid it completely. This deficiency exists in varying degrees of seriousness. Some people find they can get along on one eight-ounce glass of milk a day or even a meal, but they can't tolerate more.

If you have this problem, you should experiment to see how much of dairy products you can consume. You may be able to eat or drink enough to make your 1000- to 1500-milligram quota of calcium each day. If you can't, you should try one of the calcium-fortified foods, such as fortified orange juice, now available in most supermarkets; or you might try a supplement recommended by your doctor. Whatever your approach, be sure that you take in enough calcium each day. Those older people who consume the national average of 450 to 500 milligrams per day are in serious danger of suffering additional bone loss, and those past sixty-five need 1500 milligrams of calcium daily.

#4: THE SUPPLEMENT ISSUE

In the past, a basic principle underlying many nutrition programs has been that a proper diet should make supplements unnecessary, but recent research findings suggest that certain supplements can provide some additional health insurance. In particular, if you are a woman past the age of menopause, you should consider taking calcium supplements. Also, it's important to take in sufficient amounts of the antioxidant vitamins—especially vitamins C and E and beta-carotene, the precursor of vitamin A. (For more detail on antioxidants, see my book *Antioxidant Revolution* [Thomas Nelson, 1994.])

Antioxidants get their name from the fact that they reduce or eliminate damage caused by dangerous, out-of-control molecules that often contain oxygen. These molecules, known as free radicals, are important to the
working of the immune system. But when they are present in the body in
excessive amounts, the immune system may cease to operate properly. There
is evidence that an increase in free radicals can be caused by such factors
as stress, cigarette smoke, pollution, exposure to radiation, or certain drugs.
The result of too many free radicals may be increased cancer, heart and
vessel disease, cataracts, or emphysema. A solid and growing set of scientific
studies supports the idea that antioxidant supplements will help prevent
the spread of free radicals in the body. So I suggest that my patients include
antioxidant supplements in doses according to their age, sex, and activity
levels. The standard daily dosages are 400 IU of natural vitamin E, 1000
milligrams of vitamin C, and 25000 IU of beta carotene, but more precise
guidelines are discussed in chapter 6 of the *Antioxidant Revolution* (page 127).

Another important supplement possibility is calcium. If possible, the
diet should include the recommended 1000 to 1500 milligrams of calcium
each day. These can be selected from most dairy foods, like milk and yogurt.
For example, you can achieve your minimum calcium requirement by drinking three-and-a-half eight-ounce glasses of skim milk, or three-and-a-half
cups of nonfat yogurt, or some combination of these two foods (e.g., one cup
of yogurt and two-and-a-half glasses of skim milk). If you're lactose intoler-
ant or otherwise have trouble taking in enough dairy products to meet this
goal, you may want to consider lactose-free milk or a supplement. Here are
some guidelines:

- When they are taken alone, calcium supplements seem more
  effective in preventing loss of mass of the long, hard bones in the
  body (such as the thigh bone). They don't do as much for the
  "soft" bones of the spine or ribs.
- Women who have just gone through menopause may have to take
  estrogen with a calcium supplement to stem bone loss. See your
  doctor about this.
- Different supplements are absorbed at different rates by different
  people. The most common supplements are calcium carbonate,
  calcium phosphate, calcium gluconate, and calcium citrate. Such
  factors as the acidity of the person's stomach can affect the availability of calcium in different supplements, so it's important to
  take any calcium supplement under the supervision of your physician. Also, calcium in supplement form is always better absorbed in a fasting state—that is before, not after, meals.

- No matter what supplement you take, be sure to get adequate amounts of vitamin D. Those who train outdoors will get plenty of vitamin D from sunlight. Only about twenty minutes of sunlight daily is enough for the body to make vitamin D. If for some reason your physician prescribes a vitamin D supplement, the recommended daily dose is no more than 400 to 800 international units (IU). Note: Some calcium supplements already contain vitamin D. The objective with any supplement is to raise your daily calcium intake to the 1000 to 1500 range. Don't go above that amount.

Your doctor may determine that you need other supplements, such as iron. But unless there is a good medical reason, I would suggest limiting your intake of supplements to the types and amounts listed above. Athletes especially need to depend on long-term, healthy eating practices, not on a "quick fix" from supplements, but ultra-athletes definitely need to increase the intake of antioxidants, as recommended in *The Antioxidant Revolution.*

A note on aspirin: A widely reported study involved physicians who took one 325 milligram tablet of aspirin every other day for about five years. The researchers found a 44 percent reduction in risk of heart attacks (myocardial infarctions) in the group who took aspirin, in comparison with a group who only took a placebo.

The main benefit in reducing heart attacks occurred in those fifty years old and older. On the negative side, there was a slight increase in strokes among those who took the aspirin, but the scientists said this rise was statistically insignifcant.

My present thinking on this subject, which is in accord with a large segment of the medical community, is that "baby" aspirin tablets (80 milligrams each) should be taken every day or every other day by those who have already had a heart attack. I recommend that those who have not had a heart attack stay away from aspirin, except for the occasional pain or headache, because there are too many other possible problems with this drug. For example, there may be irritation of the stomach or intestines, or a slight increase in the risk of a hemorrhagic (bleeding) stroke.

There are other supplement-related issues that you'll probably have to check with your physician. If you have high blood pressure (hypertension), you will want to watch your consumption of salt. I wouldn't recommend that *anyone,* with or without hypertension, treat salt as a "supplement" and add it to the meal at the table.

Supplements are a controversial topic in medical and nutritional circles right now, and I've taken a rather aggressive approach by giving the green light for using a few of them in some circumstances. In making these suggestions, I'm playing it safe by assuming that many people won't quite take in the maximum amount of vitamins and minerals that will provide the greatest health benefits.

A Final Exam for Amateur Nutrition Experts: Can You Outdo the National Basketball Association Rookies?

When some rookies from the NBA came to Dallas for a seminar, our Cooper Clinic Nutrition Director, Georgia Kostas, who was a guest speaker, prepared the following questions for them. The rookies got fewer than half of the questions right—a typical performance for most people who take this test. See how you do.

Some of the questions have only one right answer; others have more than one right answer. The answers are at the end. I think you'll find that this provides not only a fun quiz, but also an educational tool to help you improve your nutritional habits.

The NBA Rookie "Best Choice" Food Quiz Fluids*

Fluids
1. Which fluid is best *after* a game?
   a) beer
   b) soft drink
   c) orange juice
   d) sports drink
   e) water

2. How much fluid do you need daily?
   a) 2 quarts (8 glasses)
   b) 3 quarts (12 glasses)
   c) 4 quarts (16 glasses)

3. Which fluid is best *during* a game?
   a) water
   b) sports drinks
   c) no water/fluid to prevent cramps

4. How much fluid is best *1 hour before* a game?
   a) ½ cup
   b) 1 cup
   c) 2 cups

*Georgia Kostas, M.P.H., R.D., Director of Nutrition, Cooper Clinic, Aerobics Center, Dallas, Texas, September 25, 1990.

Meals (low-fat, carbohydrate)

1. You are running through an airport. Which snack or food is best in each following set?

A. *(choose one)*
   a) nachos
   b) french fries
   c) soft pretzels

B. *(choose one)*
   a) chips
   b) nuts
   c) popcorn

C. *(choose one)*
   a) hot dog
   b) hamburger
   c) roast beef sandwich

D. *(choose one)*
   a) cold cut sandwich
   b) sausage biscuit
   c) turkey sandwich

E. *(choose one)*
   a) croissant
   b) biscuit
   c) bagel

F. *(choose one)*
   a) chocolate bar
   b) peanuts
   c) granola bar

2. *After* a late game, which fast food is best?
   a) hamburger
   b) pizza
   c) Mexican food

3. *Before* a game, which is best?
   a) chicken and spaghetti dinner
   b) steak dinner
   c) all liquid meal

4. *Right after* a game (in the locker room), which is best?
   a) fruit
   b) sandwich
   c) nuts

5. At Mexican restaurants, which is the best?

Appetizer
   a) nachos
   b) tortilla chips/salsa
   c) soft tortillas/salsa

Entree
   a) fajitas
   b) enchiladas
   c) tamales

Fast Food
   a) bean burrito
   b) beef burrito
   c) chicken taco

6. Which is the best *pizza?*
   a) sausage
   b) cheese
   c) pepperoni

7. Which fast food *sandwich* is best?
   a) hamburger (small)
   b) fried chicken sandwich
   c) fried fish filet sandwich

8. Which *steak* is best?
   a) rib eye
   b) filet
   c) prime rib

9. Which *dessert* is best?
   a) chocolate cake
   b) homemade cookies
   c) banana split

10. Which *bread* is best? (pick 6)
    a) cornbread
    b) whole wheat bread
    c) French bread
    d) bran muffin
    e) English muffin
    f) danish roll
    g) dinner roll
    h) bagel

11. Which *sandwich* is best:
    a) turkey
    b) roast beef
    c) ham

Body Language
1. What percent body fat is best for you?
   a) 5 to 10 percent
   b) 10 to 15 percent
   c) 15 to 20 percent

2. Which cholesterol level is best for athletic men in their 20s?
   a) less than 200
   b) less than 220
   c) less than 250

What is your cholesterol level? _____

Answers

Fluids

1. c, d, e. It's advisable to drink one quart of water and one quart of other fluids that contain carbohydrate calories and electrolytes, such as juices and sports drinks. The sugars in juices and sports drinks raise the glycogen in the muscles approximately 50 percent faster if they are consumed in the first hour after exercise.
2. c. Active athletes need at least two quarts of water and two quarts of other noncaffeinated drinks.
3. a, b. Until very recently, we thought that only water should be drunk during a game. Now, we know that sports drinks containing 5 to 10 percent sugar concentration may be even better.
4. c. Adequate hydration before a game delays fatigue.

Meals

1. A-c. B-c. C-c. D-c. E-c. F-c. Other good choices include raisins, dried fruit, cereal mix, and fresh fruit.
2. b. Half of a twelve-inch cheese pizza is lower in fat than hamburger or Mexican food.
3. a. If time permits, a solid, high-carbohydrate meal four to six hours before a game is best.
4. a. Even better would be fruit, plus yogurt, plus fruit juice. The more carbohydrates, the better!
5. Appetizer-c. Entree-a. Fast food choice-a.
6. b.
7. a.
8. b.
9. c. Although all the choices have more than 50 percent fat, the banana split has more water and potassium.
10. b, c, d, e, g, h. These are virtually fat-free.
11. a.

Body Language

1. a. Caution: This low body-fat figure is for young professional male basketball players. Over forty athletes should stick to the guidelines I've stated elsewhere: less than 18 percent for women and less than 15 percent for men. Older men and women who are not competitive athletes can still be healthy with a body fat percentage that is about 3 to 4 percent higher than these levels.
2. a. *Cholesterol level:* Only two out of 100 NBA rookies knew their cholesterol levels! By now, I hope you know yours!

$$\boxed{15}$$

HOW LONG—AND HOW WELL—
WILL YOU LIVE?

My philosophy has always been that it's better to *grow* old than to
get old. We all must age; but we don't have to age at an accelerated rate.

A major goal of this book has been to encourage the relatively inactive
person to embark on a more active life and to allow personal faith to become
the driving force that makes the program successful. Physical fitness
achieved at *any* level of activity is an essential ingredient in slowing down
the process of aging and turning life into a far more useful, enjoyable—and
independent—affair.

Great Independence from
"Squaring Off the Curve"

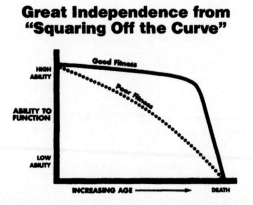

Americans are living longer than ever before, with average life expectancy exceeding seventy-five years. Yet many are not really living; they are
just existing. They have developed chronic health conditions that have
robbed them of their independence and autonomy.

The magnitude of this problem can be seen clearly in a study on
independence and aging published in the U.S. Public Health Service's *Pre-*

vention Report in October 1991. This investigation showed that in 1980, when life expectancy in the United States was nearly seventy-four years of age, the expectancy for a *healthy* life was only sixty-two years. In other words, Americans lived nearly twelve years of their life expectancy with some sort of chronic condition—such as a heart problem, joint disease, or back ailment. The condition could be expected to affect their ability to function independently and to impair their quality of life.

But such a depressing result isn't inevitable. Our goal as we grow older should be, as gerontologists say, to "square off the curve." What this means is that as you age, bodily functions can be plotted on a linear graph, with the curve dipping downward from maximum health and capacity in the younger years to a cessation of functioning at death.

For most people, there is a steady decline in physical functioning—a gradually dipping curve on the graph—which in effect leads to slow death in the last twelve years of life. During this last phase, the quality of life is poor and is characterized by dependence on others.

But those who enter their advanced years in a healthy, fit state can actually condense the time of senility or limited capacity to function into a short period, immediately prior to death. They find that, during most of life, they deteriorate very slowly until death finally overtakes them. The curve that indicates their ability to function in later life is thus "squared off." The graph line representing their ability to operate powerfully and independently stays high until the very last moment. Then, the line plunges at almost a 90-degree angle to indicate the complete loss of physical abilities at death.

But the benefits of ongoing fitness go far beyond the individual. Fitness after forty can also make you a more active parent and grandparent, reduce the costs of health care, and free your relatives to pursue their own lives, without having to worry about caring for you.

MORE ACTIVE PARENTS AND GRANDPARENTS

The fit person, with his or her additional energy, strength, endurance, and good health, is able to keep up more easily with children and grandchildren.

I'm reminded of the scene during a recent soccer season for eight- and nine-year-olds. One sixty-year-old man brought a portable chair to watch a young relative's performance—when he felt like attending at all. Yet a sixty-five-year-old grandmother walked or jogged constantly back and forth between the goals as the ball moved from one end of the field to the other. As she kept on the go, she took snapshots with her camera and cheered for her granddaughter's side.

The lesson is clear: If you're in shape, you can enjoy and assist younger family members well into your later years. If you're not, you may have to stay planted on the sidelines as a rather limited spectator.

There's also an increased sense of *togetherness* in the family that runs, swims, or otherwise works out as a group. Some of my most enjoyable times with my children and my wife have been jogs, walks, or climbs up demanding mountains. We couldn't have experienced those supreme moments of joy without being fit.

REDUCED COSTS FOR HEALTH CARE

If you pay your own health insurance costs, as business owners or sole proprietors must do, you know how burdensome it is to pay premiums and deductibles year after year for poor health. Life insurance premiums are another high-cost item for those who smoke, have high cholesterol, or otherwise are in poor health.

But the problem goes beyond the individual who has to pay to society at large. A study from the RAND Health Insurance Experiment, published in the *American Journal of Public Health* has reported that the cost to society of a sedentary lifestyle is $1900 per person. In other words, fit people subsidize the health problems of unfit people to the tune of $1900 per sedentary person over a lifetime.

Factors included in the cost analysis were such items as health insurance, sick-leave coverage, disability insurance, and group life insurance. If all those unfit people would just start on sound exercise and nutrition programs, we could greatly lower those costs through reduced health care outlays.

In one model program that has attempted to reverse the health care problem that faces society, the Mesa Corporation of Dallas and Amarillo, Texas, has instituted a fitness center and wellness program. Among other things, the corporation has significantly reduced its health care costs and has lowered absentee rates.

Specifically, Mesa's average health care cost per employee was $1,121, while the national average was $2,750. Also, Mesa exercisers averaged less than half the sick days of the national average. Finally, in the period studied, the Mesa researchers found that the medical claims of exercisers in their company averaged only $236 per year, a figure that was one-half of the $572 average annual medical claims of the non-exercisers in the company.

A FREEING OF OTHER RELATIVES

I've said a great deal about how a higher level of fitness can enable *you* to be more independent as you age. But what about your loved ones?

It's a fact of life that if you become disabled, infirm, or dependent through the process of aging, someone will have to care for you.

Who will become the caregiver? A relatively small number of the thirty million Americans over sixty-five live in nursing homes. In fact, about 9 percent live in nursing facilities at some time, another 70 percent are independent, and 21 percent rely on family members. Of course, that 30 percent in nursing homes or under the care of a relative includes a disproportionately large number of the "oldest old"—those who are in their late seventies, eighties, or older.

In most cases, the family caregivers are women. According to a study by the American Association of Retired Persons, about 31 percent of the caregivers are part of the nation's corporate management. As a result, 18 percent had lost time from work during the past six months because of problems involving the dependent relative. Also, 22 percent of the caregivers hadn't taken a vacation away from their dependent relative for at least a year.

You can begin to see the ripple effects of being in shape, as opposed to allowing your body to deteriorate with age. A lack of fitness has an impact on loved ones and society at large, not just on the sedentary individual.

On a personal note, as I look at my own prospects for a long and productive life, I only hope I can be as lucky as both my mother and father. Both of them certainly "squared off the curve."

My father, a practicing dentist in Oklahoma for some fifty years, worked all day on a Friday and died on the following Monday. He was seventy-seven years old at the time.

Ten years later, my mother, age eighty-two, voted in the presidential elections. She then went home that night and stretched out on the sofa to watch the election returns on television. She passed away sometime during the night, and we found her there on the sofa the next morning—still wearing a lapel pin that said, "I voted today."

At the time of her death, she was living in her own home, driving her own car, and operating in a totally independent manner—and what she feared worse than death was losing her independence.

As for me, I'm a lot like my parents. I want to live *fully*, up to the very last moment. If I maximize my physical potential, I know I'll be more productive at work and at home, and I believe I am more likely to be used effectively by God. Fitness that can be used as a platform to achieve personal and spiritual goals is what I want for you, as well as for myself. To achieve this goal and to "square off the curve" of your life, it's necessary to strive constantly to become stronger, to develop greater endurance, and to achieve better flexibility. Those who test their limits in such ways are more likely to taste life in all its abundance.

REFERENCES

Chapter One
  Isaiah 40:31

Chapter Two
  1 Timothy 4:8
  1 Corinthians 6:19-20

Chapter Three
  Benson, Herbert M., *Beyond the Relaxation Response* (New York: Times Books, 1984).
  Genesis 1:31
  1 Timothy 4:4
  1 Timothy 4:8
  Psalm 32:3-4
  Philippians 4:13
  James 1:6-8

Chapter Four
  Anderson, Keaven M., Ph.D., William P. Castelli, M.D., and Daniel Levy, M.D. "Cholesterol and Mortality: 30 Years of Follow-Up from the Framingham Study," *Journal of the American Medical Association,* vol. 257, no. 16, April 24, 1987, pp. 2176-2180.
  Beall, Cynthia M., Melvyn C. Goldstein, and Edward S. Feldman. "The Physical Fitness of Elderly Nepalese Farmers Residing in Rugged Mountain and Flat Terrain," *Journal of Gerontology,* vol. 40, no. 5, 1985 pp. 529-535.
  Brown, Greg, M.D., Ph.D., John J. Albers, Ph.D., Lloyd D. Fisher, Ph.D., Susan M. Schaefer, B.A., Jiin-Tarng Lin, M.D., M.P.H., Cheryl Kaplan, R.D., Xue-Qiao Zhao, M.D., Brad D. Bisson, B.S., Virginia F. Fitzpatrick, M.S., and Harold T. Dodge, M.D. "Regresson of Coronary Artery Disease as a Result of Intensive Lipid-Lowering Therapy in Men with High Levels of Apolipoprotein B," *New England Journal of Medicine,* vol. 323, no. 19, Nov. 8, 1990, pp. 1289-1298.
  Cooper, Kenneth H., J. Gerry Purdy, Steve R. White, Michael L. Pollock, and A.C. Linnerud. "Age-Fitness Adjusted Maximal Heart Rates," *Medicine Sport,* vol. 10 (Karger, Basel 1977), Institute for Aerobics Research, Dallas, TX, pp. 78-88.
  Dunn, Marian E., Ph.D. "Psychological Perspectives of Sex and Aging," *American Journal of Cardiology,* 61, 1988, pp. 1:24H-26H.
  Fiatarone, Maria A., M.D., Elizabeth C. Marks, M.S., Nancy D. Ryan, D.T., Carol N. Meredith, Ph.D., Lewis A. Lipsitz, M.D., and William J. Evans, Ph.D. "High-Intensity Strength Training in Nonagenarians," *Journal of The American Medical Association,* vol. 263, no. 22, June 13, 1990, pp. 3029-3034.
  Fiatarone, Maria A., M.D. "Strength Improvements at Any Age," *Running & FitNews,* vol. 7, no. 11, Nov. 1989, p. 1.
  Higginbotham, Michael B., M.B., Kenneth G. Morris, M.D., R. Sanders Williams, M.D., R. Edward Coleman, M.D., and Frederick R. Cobb, M.D. "Physiologic Basis for the Age-Related Decline in Aerobic Work Capacity," *American Journal of Cardiology,* 57, 1986, pp. 1374-1379.

Holloszy, John O. "Exercise, Health, and Aging: A Need for More Information," *Medicine and Science in Sports and Exercise,* vol. 15, no. 1, 1983, pp. 1–5.

Jernigan, James A., M.D., John C. Gudat, Ph.D., Jerome L. Blake, M.T., Laura Bowen, P.A.-C., and Dennis C. Lezotte, Ph.D. "Reference Values for Blood Findings in Relatively Fit Elderly Persons," *Journal of The American Geriatrics Society,* vol. 28, no. 7, 1980, p. 308.

Kasch, Fred W., Ph.D., John L. Boyer, M.D., Steven P. Van Camp, M.D., Larry S. Verity, Ph.D., and Janet P. Wallace, Ph.D. "The Effect of Physical Activity and Inactivity on Aerobic Power in Older Men (A Longitudinal Study)," *The Physician and Sportsmedicine,* vol. 18, no. 4, April 1990, p. 73.

Nash, Heyward L. "Exercising the Body to Sharpen the Mind," *The Physician and Sportsmedicine,* vol. 14, no. 4, April, 1986, p. 34.

Ornish, Dean, Shirley E. Brown, Larry W. Scherwitz, James H. Billings, William T. Armstrong, Thomas A. Ports, Sandra M. McLanahan, Richard L. Kirkeeide, Richard J. Brand, and K. Lance Gould. "Can Lifestyle Changes Reverse Coronary Heart Disease?" *The Lancet,* vol. 336, pp. 129–133.

Peitzman, Steven J., M.D., and Stanley R. Berger. "Postprandial Blood Pressure Decrease in Well Elderly Persons," *Arch Intern Med,* vol. 149, Feb. 1989, pp. 286–288.

Perkins, Kenneth A., Ph.D., Stephen R. Rapp, Ph.D., Charles R. Carlson, Ph.D., and Clinton E. Wallace, M.D., "A Behavioral Intervention to Increase Exercise among Nursing Home Residents," *The Gerontologist,* vol. 26, no. 5, 1989, p. 479.

Porterfield, Kay Marie. "A Sexual Second Wind?" *American Health,* Jan.-Feb. 1990, p. 33.

Robbins, Alan S., M.D., Laurence Z. Rubenstein, M.D., M.P.H., Karen R. Josephson, M.P.H., Barbara L. Schulman, R.N., G.N.P., Dan Osterweil, M.D., and Gilbert Fine, M.S. "Predictors of Falls Among Elderly People: Results of Two Population-Based Studies," *Arch Intern Med,* vol. 149, July 1989, pp. 1628–1633.

Rodeheffer, Richard J., M.D., Gary Gerstenblith, M.D., Lewis C. Becker, M.D., Jerome L. Fleg, M.D., Myron L. Weisfeldt, M.D., and Edward G. Lakatta, M.D. "Exercise Cardiac Output Is Maintained with Advancing Age in Healthy Human Subjects: Cardiac Dilatation and Increased Stroke Volume Compensate for a Diminished Heart Rate," *Circulation,* vol. 60, no. 2, Feb. 1984, pp. 203–213.

Sinaki, Mehrsheed, M.D. "Exercise and Osteoporosis," *Arch Phys Med Rehabil,* vol. 70, March 1989, pp. 220–229.

Stuller, Stu. "Run Long and Prosper," *Runner's World,* July 1985, p. 71.

Thompson, Keith. "Exercise Boosts Body's Clot-Busting Ability," *The Physician and Sportsmedicine,* vol. 18, no. 3, March 1990, p. 43.

Tjoa, Hong I., M.D., and Norman M. Kaplan, M.D. "Treatment of Hypertension in the Elderly," *Journal of The American Medical Association,* vol. 264, no. 8, Aug. 22/29, 1990, pp. 1015–1018.

Van Camp, Steven P., M.D., and Richard A. Peterson, Ph.D. "Cardiovascular Complications of Outpatient Cardiac Rehabilitation Programs," *Journal of The American Medical Association,* vol. 256, no. 9, Sept. 5, 1986, pp. 1160–1163.

Willis, Lee, Ronald A. Yeo, Paula Thomas, and Phillip J. Garry. "Differential Declines in Cognitive Function with Aging: The Possible Role of Health Status," *Developmental Neuropsychology,* 4(1), 1988, pp. 23–28.

Wilmore, Jack H., Ph.D. "Exercise Testing, Training, and Beta-Adrenergic Blockade," *The Physician and Sportsmedicine,* vol. 16, no. 12, Dec. 1988, p. 45.

Work, Janis A., Ph.D. "Strength Training: A Bridge to Independence for the Elderly," *The Physician and Sportsmedicine,* vol. 17, no. 11, Nov. 1989, p. 134.

Zauber, N. Peter, M.D., and Ann G. Zauber, Ph.D. "Hematologic Data of Healthy Old People," *Journal of the American Medical Association,* vol. 257, no. 16, April 24, 1987, pp. 2181–2184.

Chapter Five
1 Peter 5:7
"Aging: Can It Be Slowed?" *Business Week,* Feb. 8, 1988, p. 58.

Blair, Steven N., Patricia A. Brill, and Harold W. Kohl, III. "Physical Activity Patterns in Older Individuals," Institute for Aerobics Research, Dallas, p. 120.

Haber, P., B. Honiger, M. Klicpera, and M. Niederberger. "Effects in Elderly People 67–76 Years of Age of Three-Month Endurance Training on a Bicycle Ergometer," *European Heart Journal*, 5 (Supplement E), 1984, pp. 37–39.

Hjort Sorensen, Kirsten. "State of Health and Its Association with Death among Old People at Three-Years Follow-Up," Institute for Almen Medicin, Københavns Universitet, Juliane Maries Vej 18, DK-2100 København O, p. 121.

Hochschild, Richard, M.A. "Biological Age as a Measure of Risk," *Journal of American Society of CLU & ChFC*, Sept. 1988, p. 60.

Kavanagh, Terence, M.D., and Roy J. Shepard, M.D., Ph.d., D.P.E. "Can Regular Sports Participation Slow the Aging Process? Data on Masters Athletes," *The Physician and Sportsmedicine*, vol. 18, no. 6, June 1990, p. 94.

Shepard, John G., and Lauren C. Pacelli. "Why Your Patients Shouldn't Take Aging Sitting Down," *The Physician and Sportsmedicine*, vol. 18, no. 11, Nov. 1990, p. 83.

Stockton, William. "Can Exercise Alter the Aging Process?" *The New York Times*, Nov. 28, 1988.

Strovas, Jane. "Chronic Illness Need Not Deter Elderly Exercisers," *The Physician and Sportsmedicine*, vol. 18, no. 2, Feb. 1990, p. 20.

"U.S. Preventive Services Task Force." (Reprint) *Journal of the American Medical Association*, vol. 261, June 23/30, 1989, p. 3588.

Westcott, Wayne L., Ph.D. "Slowing Down the Clock," *Cycling & Fitness*, p. 13.

Chapters Six, Seven, and Eight
Psalm 18:32–33
The main sources for the programs and other materials in these exercise chapters are my own clinical testing and research, which I have conducted during the last three decades in the United States Air Force, at the Cooper Clinic in Dallas, and at the Cooper Institute for Aerobics Research in Dallas.

Chapter Nine
Brant, John, "Master of Time," *Runner's World*, Dec. 1988, p. 29.

Lane, Nancy E., M.D., Daniel A. Bloch, Ph.D., Henry H. Jones, M.D., William H. Marshall, Jr., M.D., Peter D. Wood, Ph.D., and James F. Fries, M.D., "Long-Distance Running, Bone Density, and Osteoarthritis," *Journal of The American Medical Association*, vol. 255, no. 9, March 7, 1986, pp. 1147–1151.

Mason, Margaret. "Body & Soul: 50-Plus and Running," *The Washington Post*, April 16, 1990.

Mueller, Herman. "Annabel Marsh—Can-Do Lady," *Fifty-Plus Bulletin*, Dec. 1990, p. 1.

"No Age Limit to Exercise Benefits," *Running & FitNews* (Interview with Ronald M. Lawrence, M.D.; also *Journal of the American Medical Association*, vol. 252, no. 5, Aug. 3, 1984, pp. 645–649), Nov. 1984, p. 1.

Chapter Ten
Cooper, Bob. "Helen Klein: Grand Slam Grandma Keeps On Improving," *Ultrarunning*, Nov. 1990, p. 34.

"Do Swimmers Age Faster Than Runners?" *Runner's World*, Aug. 1989, p. 6.

Higdon, Hal. "Double Your Endurance," *Runner's World*, Dec. 1990.

"Marczak Top Age-Graded Runner at Twin Cities," *National Masters News*, issue 147, Nov. 1990, p. 1.

"19 Years, 100,000 Miles: An M.D. Runs for Health, Solitude, and Knowledge," *American Medical News*, July 29, 1988, p. 1.

Parker Jr., John L., ed., "And Then the Vulture Eats You; Ultramarathons: Journeys of Discovery," Tallahassee, FL: (Cedarwinds Pub. Co., 1991).

Pereira, Joseph. "He Paints Still Lifes but John Kelley, 83, Is Still on the Move," *The Wall Street Journal*, March 26, 1991, p. 1.

"Training the Older Athlete; Part II—Practical Considerations," *NSCA Journal,* vol. 10, no. 6, 1988, p. 10.

Tymm, Mike. "The Effects of Motivation and Adaptation on the Aging Curve," *Runner's World,* July 1989, p. 6.

Walker, J.M., T.C. Floud, G. Fein, C. Cavness, R. Lualhati, and I. Feinberg, "Effects and Exercise on Sleep," Veterans Administration Hospital, and University of California, San Francisco, CA 94121.

"Who Holds the Most Running Records?" *Running Times,* Aug. 1985, p. 14.

Chapter Eleven

Baylor, Ann M., and Waneen W. Spirduso. "Systematic Aerobic Exercise and Components of Reaction Time in Older Women," Department of Kinesiology and Health Education and Institute for Neurological Sciences Reserach, The University of Texas at Austin, p. 121.

Black Sandler, Rivka, Ph.D. "Muscle Strength Assessments and the Prevention of Osteoporosis," *The American Geriatrics Society,* 1989, pp. 1192–1197.

Cinque, Chris. "Women's Strength Training: Lifting the Limits of Aging?" *The Physician and Sportsmedicine,* vol. 18, no. 8, Aug. 1990, p. 123.

Conrad Johnston Jr., C., M.D., and Charles Slemenda, D.P.H. "Osteoporosis: An Overview," *The Physician and Sportsmedicine,* vol. 15, no. 11, Nov. 1987, p. 65.

"Estrogen Use Prevents Postmenopausal Hip Fracture," *Internal Medicine Alert,* vol. 9, no. 22, Nov. 30, 1987, p. 85.

Foster, V.L., G.J.E. Hume, A.L. Dickinson, S.J. Chatfield, and W.C. Byrnes. "The Reproducibility of VO_{2max}, Ventilatory, and Lactate Thresholds in Elderly Women," *Medicine and Science in Sports and Exercise,* American College of Sports Medicine, vol. 18, no. 4, 1986, p. 425.

Halioua, Lydia, and John J.B. Anderson. "Lifetime Calcium Intake and Physical Activity Habits: Independent and Combined Effects on the Radial Bone of Healthy Premenopausal Caucasian Women," *American Journal of Clinical Nursing,* vol. 49, 1989, pp. 534–541.

Matthews, Karen, Ph.D., Elaine Meilahn, M.P.H., Lewis H. Kuller, M.D., Dr. P.H., Sheryl F. Kelsey, Ph.D., Arlene W. Caggiula, Ph.D., and Rena R. Wing, Ph.D. "Menopause and Risk Factors for Coronary Heart Disese," *New England Journal of Medicine,* vol. 321, no. 10, 1989, pp. 641–646.

McElmurry, Beverly J., Ed.D., F.A.A.N., and Susan J. LiBrizzi, R.N., M.S. "The Health of Older Women," *Nursing Clinics of North America,* vol. 21, no. 1, March 1986, pp. 161–171.

"New Study Confirms Benefit of Cyclical Etidronate for Postmenopausal Osteoporosis," *Internal Medicine Alert,* vol. 12, no. 14, July 29, 1990, p. 53.

Portz-Shovlin, Eileen, "The Human Race," *Runner's World,* Dec. 1990, p. 94.

"Prevention and Treatment of Postmenopausal Osteoporosis," *The Medical Letter,* vol. 29, issue 746, Aug. 14, 1987, p. 75.

Richelson, Linda S., M.P.H., Heinz W. Wahner, M.D., L.J. Melton III, M.D., and B. Lawrence Riggs, M.D. "Relative Contributions of Aging and Estrogen Deficiency to Postmenopausal Bone Loss," *New England Journal of Medicine,* vol. 311, no. 20, 1984, pp. 1272–1275.

Smith, Everett L., Ph.D. "How Exercise Helps Prevent Osteoporosis," *The Active Woman,* p. 51.

Wardlaw, Gordon, Ph.D., R.D. "The Effects of Diet and Life-style on Bone Mass in Women," *Journal of The American Dietetic Association,* vol. 88, Jan. 1988, p. 17.

Watts, Nelson B., M.D., Steven T. Harris, M.D., Harry K. Genant, M.D., Richard D. Wasnich, M.D., Paul D. Miller, M.D., Rebecca D. Jackson, M.D., Angelo A. Licata, M.D., Ph.D., Philip Ross, Ph.D., Grattan C. Woodson, III, M.D., Melissa J. Yanover, M.D., W. Jerry Mysiw, M.D., Larry Kohse, M.D., M. Bhaskar Rao, M.D., Peter Steiger, Ph.D., Bradford Richmond, M.D., and Charles H. Chesnut, III, M.D. "Intermittent Cyclical Etidronate Treatment of Postmenopausal Osteoporosis," *New England Journal of Medicine,* vol. 323, no. 2, July 12, 1990, pp. 73–79.

"Will Exercise Help Keep Women Away from Oncologists—or Obstetricians?" *Journal of The American Medical Association,* vol. 259, no. 12, March 25, 1988, p. 1769.

"Women and Heart Disease," *HeartCorps,* vol. 2, no. 2, Oct. 1989, p. 50.

Chapter Twelve

"ACSM Guidelines for Fitness Updated," *Running & FitNews,* vol. 8, no. 7, July 1990, p. 1.

Albohm, Marjorie J. "Musculoskeletal Injuries," *Aerobic Dance-Exercise Instructor Manual,* JDEA Foundation, p. 269.

" 'Born' as a Runner at 67, California Physician Still Runs for Health, Glory," *American Medical News,* June 28/July 5, 1985, p. 3.

Brody, Jane E. "Water Aerobics: A Low-Risk Medium for Exercise That Offers a Broad Range of Benefits," *New York Times,* p. B16.

"Chronically Sick People Also Benefit from Exercise," *Running & FitNews,* vol. 8, no. 6, June 1990, p. 1.

Cooper, Kenneth H., M.D., M.P.H. "Fitness, Coronary Risk Factors, and Preventive Medicine." Address presented to American Life Insurance Association Medical Section Annual Meeting, Colorado Springs, CO, June 13, 1974.

Crittenden, John. "Fitness a Year-Round Job for Athletes," *New York Times,* March 11, 1991.

DeBenedette, Valerie. "Stair Machines: The Truth about This Fitness Fad," *The Physician and Sportsmedicine,* vol. 18, no. 6, June 1990, p. 131.

Dominquez, Dr. Richard. "Warning: These Exercises Can Be Dangerous to Your Health!" *Total Body Training,* p. 51.

"Female Factor, The," *University of California, Berkeley Wellness Letter,* vol. 4, issue 6, March 1988, p. 1.

Frankel, Lawrence J., and Betty Byrd Richard. *Be Alive As Long as You Live,* (Charleston, WVA: Preventicare Publications, 1977).

Grimby, Gunnar. "Physical Activity and Muscle Training in the Elderly," *Acta Med Scand. Suppl.* from the Department of Rehabilitation Medicine, Göteborgs Universitet, Göteborg, Sweden, 711, 1986, pp. 233–237.

Higdon, Hal. "Forever Fit," *Wellness,* Oct. 1986, p. 11.

Higdon, Hal. *The Masters Running Guide,* 1990.

"Ingrid Kristiansen." *Runner's World,* Feb. 1988, p. 55.

Monahan, Terry. "From Activity to Eternity," *The Physician and Sportsmedicine,* vol. 14, no. 6, June 1986, p. 156.

Paffenbarger, Jr., Ralph S., M.D., Dr. P.H., Robert T. Hyde, M.A., Alvin L. Wing, M.B.A., and Chung-Cheng Hsieh, Sc.D. "Physical Activity, All-Cause Mortality, and Longevity of College Alumni," *New England Journal of Medicine,* 1986, vol. 314, no. 10, pp. 605–613.

Phillips, Greg, M.S. "Has the Bend Been Banned?" *Aerobics and Fitness,* Jan./Feb. 1987.

"Physical Exercise: An Important Factor for Health," *The Physician and Sportsmedicine,* vol. 18, no. 3, March 1990, p. 155.

Posner, Joel D., M.D., Kevin M. Gorman, B.S., Howard S. Klein, M.D., and Asher Woldow, M.D. "Exercise Capacity in the Elderly," *American Journal of Cardiology,* vol. 57, 1986, pp. 52C-58C.

Simon, Harvey B., M.D. "Physician-al Fitness: Setting an Example," *The Physician and Sportsmedicine,* vol. 17, no. 10, Oct. 1989, p. 45.

"Strength Connection, The: How to Build Strength and Improve the Quality of Your Life," Institute for Aerobics Reserach, Dallas, TX, 1990.

Van Camp, Steven P., M.D., and John L. Boyer, M.D. "Exercise Guidelines for the Elderly" (Part 2 of 2), *The Physician and Sportsmedicine,* vol. 17, no. 5, May 1989, p. 83.

Witherell, Mary. "Players in Their 80s Going Strong in 90s." *New York Times,* Jan. 28, 1991.

Work, Janis A., Ph.D. "Strength Training: A Bridge to Independence for the Elderly," *The Physician and Sportsmedicine,* vol. 17, no. 11, Nov. 1989, p. 134.

Chapter Thirteen
Blair, Steven N., P.E.D., Harold W. Kohl III, M.S.P.H., Ralph S. Paffenbarger, Jr., M.D., Dr., Ph.D., Debra G. Clark, M.S., Kenneth H. Cooper, M.D., M.P.H., Larry W. Gibbons, M.D., M.P.H. "Physical Fitness and All-Cause Mortality: A Prospective Study of Healthy Men and Women," *Journal of The American Medical Association,* vol. 262, no. 17, Nov. 3, 1989, p. 2395.

Brody, Jane E. "Study Indicates Moderate Exercise Can Add Years to a Person's Life," *New York Times,* March 6, 1986, p. 1.

Colsher, Patricia L., Ph.D., Robert B. Wallace, M.D., Paul R. Pomrehn, M.D., Andrew Z. LaCroix, Ph.D., Joan Cornoni-Huntley, Ph.D., Dan Blazer, M.D., Ph.D., Paul A. Scherr, Ph.D., Lisa Berkman, Ph.D., and Charles H. Hennekens, M.D. "Demographic and Health Characteristics of Elderly Smokers: Result From Established Populations for Epidemiologic Studies of the Edlerly," *American Journal of Preventive Medicine,* 1990, vol. 6(2), pp. 61–70.

"Coronary Heart Disease Attributable to Sedentary Lifestyle—Selected States, 1988," *Morbidity and Mortality Weekly Report,* Centers for Disease Control, vol. 39, no. 32, Aug. 1, 1990, p. 1.

"Exercise Alone Cuts Blood Pressure in Study." *New York Times,* June 11, 1991, p. c2.

"Growth Hormone for the Elderly?" *New England Journal of Medicine,* July 5, 1990, p. 52.

Hardy, Cheryl, Ph.D., Clinton Wallace, M.D., Tawfiq Khansur, M.D., Ralph B. Vance, M.D., J. Tate Thigpen, M.D., and Lodovico Balducci, M.D. "Nutrition, Cancer, and Aging: An Annotated Review: II. Cancer Cachexia and Aging," *Journal of the American Geriatric Society,* vol. 34, 1986, pp. 219–228.

Klevay, Leslie, M., M.D., S.D., in Hyg. "Ischemic Heart Disease: A Major Obstacle to Becoming Old," *Clinics in Geriatric Medicine,* vol. 3, no. 2, May 1987, p. 361.

Manson, JoAnn E., M.D., Meir J. Stampfer, M.D., Charles H. Hennekens, M.D., Walter C. Willett, M.D. "Body Weight and Longevity: A Reassessment," *Journal of the American Medical Association,* vol. 257, 1987, pp. 353–358.

"Metabolic Rate Stays High After Exercise," *Running & FitNews,* vol. 7, no. 5, May 1989, p. 1.

Rudman, Daniel, M.D., Axel G. Feller, M.D., Hoskote S. Nagraj, M.D., Gregory A. Gergans, M.D., Pardee Y. Lalitha, M.D., Allen F. Goldberg, D.D.S., Robert A. Schlenker, Ph.D., Lester Cohn, M.D., Inge W. Rudman, B.S., and Dale E. Mattson, Ph.D. "Effects of Human Growth Hormone in Men over 60 Years Old," *New England Journal of Medicine,* vol. 323, no. 1, July 5, 1990, pp. 1–6.

Tanji, Jeffrey L., M.D. "Hypertension: Part 2: The Role of Medication," *The Physician and Sportsmedicine,* vol. 18, no. 8, Aug. 1990, p. 87.

Thomas, Paula D., Philip J. Garry, and James S. Goodwin, "Morbidity and Mortality in an Initially Healthy Elderly Sample: Findings After Five Years of Follow-Up," *Age and Aging,* vol. 15, 1986, pp. 105–110.

Thompson, Paul D., M.D. "The Benefits and Risks of Exercise Training in Patients with Chronic Coronary Artery Disease," *Journal of the American Medical Association,* vol. 259, no. 10, March 11, 1988, p. 1537.

Welin, Lennart, M.D., Ph.D., Kurt Svardsudd, M.D., Ph.D., Lars Wilhelmsen, M.D., Ph.D., Bo Larsson, M.D., Ph.D., and Gosta Tibblin, M.D., Ph.D. "Analysis of Risk Factors for Stroke in a Cohort of Men Born in 1913," *New England Journal of Medicine,* vol. 317, no. 9, Aug. 27, 1987, pp. 521–526.

York, Elihu, M.D., M.P.H., Robert E. Mitchell, M.D., and Ashton Graybiel, M.D. "Cardiovascular Epidemiology, Exercise, and Health: 40-Year Follow-Up of the U.S. Navy's '1000 Aviators,'" *Aviation, Space and Environmental Medicine,* June 1986, p. 597.

Chapter Fourteen
Anderson, Keaven M., Ph.D., William P. Castelli, M.D., and Daniel Levy, M.D. "Cholesterol and Mortality: 30 Years of Follow-Up from the Framingham Study," *Journal of The American Medical Association,* vol. 257, pp. 2176–2180.

"Breast Cancer," *Nutrition Action Health Letter,* March 1988, p. 1.

"Council on Scientific Affairs, Dietary Fiber and Health," *Journal of The American Medical Association,* vol. 262, no. 4, 1989, pp. 542–546.

Evans, William J., and Carol N. Meredith. "Exercise and Nutrition in the Elderly," USDA Nutrition Research Center on Aging, Tufts Univ., Boston, MA, p. 120.

Marcus, Robert. "Calcium Intake and Skeletal Integrity: Is There a Critical Relationship?" *The Journal of Nutrition,* vol. 117, Nov. 17, 1986, p. 631.

Rothschild, Peter R., M.D., Ph.D., and Zane Baranowski, C.N. *Free Radicals, Stress, and Antioxidant Enzymes,* second revised ed., 1990.

Rothstein, Morton, "Biochemical Studies of Aging," *C&EN,* August 11, 1986, p. 26.

Schneider, Edward L., M.D., and John D. Reed, Jr., B.S. "Life Extension," The National Institute on Aging, Bethesda, MD, p. 1150.

Steering Committee of the Physicians' Health Study Research Group. "Final Report on the Aspirin Component of the Ongoing Physicians' Health Study," *New England Journal of Medicine,* vol. 321, no. 3, July 20, 1989, pp. 129–135.

"Study Reinforces Salt's Tie to Blood Pressure," *New York Times,* April 7, 1991, p. 23.

"Synthetic Calcitonin for Postmenopausal Osteoporosis," *The Medical Letter,* vol. 27, issue 690, June 21, 1985, p. 1.

Young, Frank E., M.D., Ph.D., Stuart L. Nightingale, M.D., and Robert A. Temple, M.D. "The Preliminary Report of the Findings of the Aspirin Component of the Ongoing Physicians' Health Study," *Journal of the American Medical Association,* vol. 259, no. 21, June 3, 1988, p. 3158.

Chapter Fifteen

Blumenthal, James A., Ph.D., Charles F. Emergy, Ph.D., Margaret A. Walsh, M.S., David R. Cox, Ph.D., Cynthia M. Kuhn, Ph.D., Redford B. Williams, M.D., and R. Sanders Williams, M.D. "Exercise Training in Healthy Type A Middle-Aged Men: Effects on Behavioral and Cardiovascular Responses," *Psychosomatic Medicine,* vol. 50, 1988, pp. 418–433.

Clarke, Sir Cyril, K.B.E., M.D., F.R.C.P., F.R.S. "Increased Longevity In Man," *Journal of the Royal College of Physicians of London,* vol. 20, no. 2, April 1986, p. 122.

Fox, Bernard H., Ph.D. "Depressive Symptoms and Risk of Cancer," *Journal of The American Medical Association,* vol. 262, no. 9, Sept. 1, 1989, p. 1231.

"Health Care: Americans Seek Fundamental Change," *The Johns Hopkins Medical Letter,* vol. 1, issue 3, May 1989, p. 1.

Hlatky, Mark A., M.D., Robin E. Boineau, M.A., Michael B. Higginbotham, M.B., Kerry L. Lee, Ph.D., Daniel B. Mark, M.D., M.P.H., and David B. Pryor, M.D. "A Brief Self-Administered Questionnaire to Determine Functional Capacity (The Duke Activity Status Index), *American Journal of Cardiology,* Sept. 15, 1989, pp. 651–654.

Keeler, Emmett B., Ph.D., Willard G. Manning, Ph.D., Joseph P. Newhouse, Ph.D., Elizabeth M. Sloss, Ph.D., and Jeffrey Wasserman, M.A. "The External Costs of a Sedentary Lifestyle," *American Journal of Public Health,* vol. 79, no. 8, Aug. 1989, pp. 975–981.

Kovar, Mary Grace, Dr. P.H., Gerry Hendershot, Ph.D., and Evelyn Mathis. "Older People in the United States Who Receive Help with Basic Activities of Daily Living," *American Journal of Public Health,* vol. 79, no. 6, 1989, p. 778.

Ostrow, Andrew C., and David A. Dzewaltowski. "Older Adults' Perceptions of Physical Activity Participation Based on Age-Role and Sex-Role Appropriateness," *Research Quarterly for Exercise and Sport,* vol. 57, no. 9, 1986, pp. 167–169.

Pickett, George, M.D., M.P.H., and William F. Bridgers, M.D. "Prevention, Declining Mortality Rates, and the Cost of Medicare," *American Journal of Preventive Medicine,* vol. 3, no. 2, pp. 76–80.

"Retiree Wellness Not 'Too Little Too Late,'" *Worksite Wellness Works,* Wellness Councils of America, Aug. 1990, p. 1.

Sallis, James F., Ph.D., and Philip R. Nader, M.D. "Family Exercise: Designing a Program to Fit Everyone," *The Physician and Sportsmedicine,* vol. 18, no. 9, Sept. 1990, p. 130.

INDEX

ABOUT THE AUTHOR

Kenneth H. Cooper, M.D., M.P.H., is the author of *Aerobics, Controlling Cholesterol, Dr. Kenneth H. Cooper's Antioxidant Revolution, Advanced Nutritional Therapies,* and other best-selling books with combined sales of over twenty-eight million copies worldwide.

Dr. Cooper coined the term "aerobics" in 1968 and has received worldwide recognition for his contributions to health and fitness. In 1970, he founded the Cooper Institute for Aerobics Research, a medical facility that offers comprehensive physical evaluation, counseling, and recommendations for attaining and maintaining healthy lifestyles.

Dr. Cooper's memberships include the American Medical Association, the Texas Medical Association, and the Dallas Medical Society. He recently received the C. Everett Koop Award, honoring him for his distinguished advocacy of health and wellness.

Dr. Cooper currently lives with his wife and family in Dallas, Texas.